The SA
Transiti

MW01106514

David B. Renton • Peter Nau
Denise W. Gee
Editors

The SAGES Manual
Transitioning to Practice

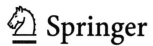 Springer

Editors
David B. Renton
The Ohio State University
Division of General Surgery
Columbus, OH, USA

Peter Nau
University of Iowa Hospitals
  and Clinics
Iowa City, IA, USA

Denise W. Gee
Massachusetts General Hospital
Division of General and
  Gastrointestinal Surgery
Boston, MA, USA

ISBN 978-3-319-51396-6   ISBN 978-3-319-51397-3   (eBook)
DOI 10.1007/978-3-319-51397-3

Library of Congress Control Number: 2017934219

Printed on acid-free paper

This Springer imprint is published by Springer Nature
The registered company is Springer International Publishing AG
The registered company address is: Gewerbestrasse 11, 6330 Cham, Switzerland

Foreword

Success in the surgical field depends on many factors. The most important factors are skill and knowledge in the operating room and experience in taking care of patients. Our residency programs do an excellent job in teaching residents and fellows these skills. The other half of success comes from excelling in the business of being a surgeon. The average time a surgeon spends at their first job coming out of training has dropped to 2 years. This manual is aimed at educating those entering the surgical job market to the business side of being a surgeon. Our goal is to increase the knowledge of those who are seeking a job and help them understand the environment they are entering, and maximize their chances of success.

Contents

Contributors

Rajesh Aggarwal, M.B.B.S., M.A., Ph.D., F.R.C.S. Department of Surgery, Faculty of Medicine, McGill University, Montreal, QC, Canada

Steinberg Centre for Simulation and Interactive Learning, Faculty of Medicine, McGill University, Montreal, QC, Canada

Maria S. Altieri, M.D. Department of Surgery, Stony Brook University Medical Center, Stony Brook, NY, USA

Erin Bresnahan, B.A. Icahn School of Medicine at Mount Sinai, New York, NY, USA

Sara E. Martin del Campo, M.D., M.S. Center for Minimally Invasive Surgery, The Ohio State University Wexner Medical Center, Columbus, OH, USA

Allison Farris, M.D. Department of Surgery, Carilion Health System, Roanoke, VA, USA

Denise W. Gee, M.D. Massachusetts General Hospital, Division of General and Gastrointestinal Surgery, Boston, MA, USA

Jon C. Gould, M.D. Department of Surgery, Medical College of Wisconsin, Milwaukee, WI, USA

Valerie Halpin, M.D. Weight and Diabetes Institute, Legacy Good Samaritan Hospital, Portland, OR, USA

Brian P. Jacob, M.D. Department of Surgery, Mount Sinai Health System, New York, NY, USA

Anjali S. Kumar, M.D., M.P.H. Department of Surgery, Virginia Mason Medical Center, Seattle, WA, USA

COL. Robert B. Lim, M.D., F.A.C.S., F.A.S.M.B.S. Department of Surgery, Tripler Army Medical Center, Honolulu, HI, USA

Aaron M. Lipskar, M.D., F.A.A.P., F.A.C.S. Division of Pediatric Surgery, Hofstra Northwell School of Medicine, Cohen Children's Medical Center, New Hyde Park, NY, USA

Susan D. Moffatt-Bruce, M.D., Ph.D., F.A.C.S. Department of General Surgery, The Ohio State University Wexner Medical Center, Columbus, OH, USA

Division of Thoracic Surgery, The Ohio State University Wexner Medical Center, Columbus, OH, USA

Adam C. Nelson, M.D. Department of General Surgery, Mount Sinai Hospital, New York, NY, USA

Michelle C. Nguyen, M.D. Department of General Surgery, The Ohio State University Wexner Medical Center, Columbus, OH, USA

Division of Thoracic Surgery, The Ohio State University Wexner Medical Center, Columbus, OH, USA

Charles Paget, B.S., M.D. Department of Surgery, Carilion Clinic Virginia Tech School of Medicine, Roanoke, VA, USA

Mark Pedersen, M.D. Department of Surgery, University of Iowa Hospitals and Clinics, Iowa City, IA, USA

Rebecca P. Petersen, M.D., M.S. Department of Surgery University of Washington, Seattle, WA, USA

Aurora D. Pryor, M.D. Division of Bariatric, Foregut, and Advanced Gastrointestinal Surgery, Department of Surgery, Health Science Center T18-040, Stony Brook Medicine, Stony Brook, NY, USA

David B. Renton, M.D., M.S.P.H., F.A.C.S. Department of Surgery, The Ohio State University Wexner Medical Center, Columbus, OH, USA

Center for Minimally Invasive Surgery, The Ohio State University Wexner Medical Center, Columbus, OH, USA

Don J. Selzer, M.D., M.S. Associate Professor, Chief, Division of General Surgery, Department of Surgery, Indiana University School of Medicine

Vlad V. Simianu, M.D., M.P.H. Surgical Outcomes Research Center, University of Washington, Seattle, WA, USA

Department of Surgery University of Washington, Seattle, WA, USA

Pritam Singh, M.B.B.S., M.A., M.R.C.S. Division of Surgery, Department of Surgery & Cancer, Imperial College London & West Midlands Deanery, London, UK

Prashant Sinha, M.D., F.A.C.S. NYU Langone Medical Center, New York, NY, USA

Dimitrios Stefanidis, M.D., Ph.D., F.A.C.S. Department of Surgery, Indiana University, Indianapolis, Indiana, USA

David S. Strosberg, M.D. Department of Surgery, The Ohio State University Wexner Medical Center, Columbus, OH, USA

Yulia Zak, M.D. Assistant Professor, Department of Surgery, Icahn School of Medicine at Mount Sinai, New York, NY, USA

Stanley Zagorski, M.D., F.A.C.S. Conemaugh Memorial Medical Center, Johnstown, PA

Part I

Chapter 1
Finding a Job—Employment Services, Word of Mouth, Job Boards

Aaron M. Lipskar

Introduction

After many years of medical school, the residency match process, general surgery residency training, research fellowships, and additional fellowship match processes and training programs, you are ready and excited to take care of surgical patients both in and out of the operating room. You are ambitious and idealistic, ready to emerge from all of those grueling years to finally be a "surgeon." The training of a surgeon, however, rarely focuses on life after residency. And this life after residency starts with your first job.

Furthermore, there is startling data regarding dissatisfaction physicians in general often have with their first jobs. In fact, approximately 50% of physicians change jobs within their first 2 years, and the most common reason for this is a mismatch in expectations and practice culture [1, 2].

The goal of this section is to prepare the surgical trainee in his or her final years of training for the daunting task of navi-

A.M. Lipskar, M.D., F.A.A.P., F.A.C.S. (✉)
Division of Pediatric Surgery, Hofstra Northwell School
of Medicine, Cohen Children's Medical Center,
269-01 76th Ave, CH158, New Hyde Park, NY 11040, USA
e-mail: alipskar@northwell.edu

© Springer International Publishing AG 2017
D.B. Renton et al. (eds.), *The SAGES Manual Transitioning to Practice*, DOI 10.1007/978-3-319-51397-3_1

3

gating the surgical job market in order to maximize the odds of finding a job that fits one's expectations. Later chapters in this manual will cover both the process of choosing a job as well as salary and contract negotiations. In this chapter, however, the focus will be on the first step of the job hunt, finding a job.

Creating Your Personal Inventory

This process starts with the difficult challenge of prioritization and creation of a personal inventory (Table 1.1) [3]. For many surgical trainees, this is the first time you need to focus on your own goals and priorities rather than the goals and priorities of your patients, attendings, and training programs/institutions. For some this will be a process of self-reflection, but for many this process intimately involves the input and guidance from an inner circle of mentors, friends, and family.

There will often be conflicts when you are creating this inventory: conflicts between location and job, job and opportunity, income and lifestyle, as well as many others. Embrace these conflicts and try to honestly answer the critical questions of what you are looking for. The goal of this step of the process should be to create a "mission-statement" for yourself that details the motivations, methods, and goals for the 2-, 5-, and 10-year benchmarks. Clinical interests, personal interests, leadership goals, roles in education, and research aspirations should all be addressed. Stretch goals should be

TABLE 1.1 The creation of a personal inventory aids in framing an upcoming job search

Creating a personal inventory	
Family	Culture/religion
Geography	Diversity
Income	Recognition
Autonomy	Career potential
Call	Research
Education	Academic advancement

identified, focusing on what achievements will set you apart. These can include clinical expertise, global health, academic promotion, innovations, publications, grants, administrative promotion, as well as others. You should attempt to characterize these goals as either flexible or nonnegotiable.

Creating your personal inventory and "mission-statement" is probably the hardest part of the transition from trainee to surgeon and will change every time you are faced with an opportunity to search for jobs again in your career. Once you have thought over the basic aspects of your inventory and created your "mission-statement" you will be better prepared to start looking for job opportunities.

Matching What You Want with What Exists

Once some of the questions of your personal inventory are resolved, the real job search should begin 12–24 months prior to the completion of your training. It is important to have a basic understanding of what types of jobs are out there. Many people simplify surgical jobs into being academic or nonacademic. While it is certainly more complicated than that, if you aspire to have an "academic" career, it is important to understand what that means to you: do you want to be a clinical surgeon with academic interests or do you want to primarily be a researcher? These academic and nonacademic aspirations are essential to understand as you begin to look at what kinds of jobs are out there.

In general, there are four types of practices: academic, hospital-employed, private practice group, and private practice solo [3]. The American College of Surgeons describes these types of practices somewhat differently: private practice, academic medicine, institutional practice, as well as government and uniformed services [4]. One of the major differences in these practices is for whom you will be working, and The American College of Surgeons released a document in 2012 titled "Surgeons as Institutional Employees" that outlines many of these differences. Below is a brief overview of some of the major differences between the diverse surgical job opportunities.

Private practice opportunities focus on patient care and often provide more professional independence and freedom. The surgeon is free to decide the organization of his or her practice, as well as the hours, the hospitals in which the surgeon practices, and the type of patients that are attracted. These opportunities require business management skills and the responsibility to provide the surgeon's own employment benefits. Academic medicine on the other hand combines teaching, patient care, and research. These opportunities suit surgeons interested in a broad exposure and allow surgeons to focus on research and become part of a research community. Institutional practice opportunities offer full-time practice that is directly affiliated with a particular hospital or clinic. Emphasis is placed exclusively on patient care but the option of combining care with research and education can exist. For more information on the different types of practices as outlined by The American College of Surgeons, one can refer to their website, https://www.facs.org/education/resources/medical-students/faq/job-description   - sthash.5Sh1zi2s.dpuf.

Understanding these differences is essential in order to align your personal inventory and mission statement with realistic goals. When you have a sense of which type of practice matches what you are looking for, you are ready to actually start looking for a job.

Finding Job Opportunities

Many trainees starting the job hunt begin by looking at journal ads and governing organizations' websites. These resources, while not all-inclusive, should not be overlooked. Journals often have some job opportunities listed and representing organizations' websites are excellent places to start looking. Examples of these websites include The American College of Surgeons (http://www.facs.org/jobs), Society of American Gastrointestinal and Endoscopic Surgeons (http://

www.sages.org/jobs), as well as many specialty organizations' websites. It should be noted that many but not all of these resources require membership to the organization.

Unfortunately, the majority of job opportunities are not advertised [5]. It is therefore critical to network early and often. Networking starts locally but needs to occur on a broader scale. While there are both recruitment firms and career counselors that can be utilized (for either a contingency fee or direct payment, respectively), the majority of surgical trainees finishing their training forego these resources and network "on their own." A simple way to start the networking process is to engage local surgeons and mentors at your home institution. Local, regional, and national conferences are priceless in networking opportunities. Ask attendings that you know to introduce you to people at these conferences and meetings. Very often job opportunities are found by these "word-of-mouth" methods. The clearer your vision and inventory, the more functional this kind of networking can be.

Lastly, the idea of reaching out on your own to jobs that are desirable should not be overlooked, even if they are not actively or publicly recruiting. An e-mail or phone call from you or your program director/department head can go a long way and is often the way surgical jobs are found.

Once you have identified prospective employers, your initial contact will usually be in the form of a short letter of interest along with a CV. It is crucial that your CV is organized and accurate. There are many resources that can assist you in preparing a CV that is ready to show to prospective employers. If the prospective employer is interested in interviewing you, they will often contact you for a short phone conversation and then set up a first interview.

The Interview Process

The first interview is often a full-day event where you will meet many people. You should remember that the primary goal is to gather as much information about the opportunity and at the same time make a favorable impression [6]. It is critical to determine whether the job being offered is the opportunity for which you are looking or simply an available position. Developing a mental checklist of qualities that are of paramount importance can help frame the day and your interactions. Do their expectations and vision of your career path match your mission statement? Is there enough clinical demand to support your practice? Is there adequate research or clinical support to be successful? Is the geographical location acceptable for you and/or your spouse? You should be confident and professional while at the same time being ready to answer and ask questions. Be transparent about your goals and clinical interests. This set of interviews is the time to determine whether your career aspirations are compatible with the job that is being offered. A big mistake to avoid is bringing up salary at a first interview. These questions should be saved for later conversations. Lastly, you should look around carefully. Look at the physical structure and observe the happiness of the staff and partners in the group. As Yogi Berra so famously said, "You can observe a lot from just watching..." [7]

End your first interview with a clear communication regarding follow-up, send a thank-you note, and if your gut tells you that this is a good opportunity, set up a second interview. At the second interview you should bring your family and this is the time to really look at the geography, social aspects, and financial/benefits aspects of the opportunity. This involves taking part in tough conversations that many surgical trainees are poorly prepared to discuss. Later sections of this manual will deal with contract, salary, and benefits. Ultimately though, the second interview is the time to ensure that the job and environment match your goals that you outlined when you started this process.

Ready to Choose

Hopefully at this point in the job search process you have some potential employment options and are ready to start the next difficult part of the process, choosing a job. This, as well as the various components of salary structure, benefits, and contract negotiations, will be covered in the ensuing chapters.

Editor's Note

Finding a job can be a daunting task when done for the first time (and any time after that). We wanted to get the perspective of a physician recruiter. This is an individual who hospitals and physicians contract with to help match their opportunities with surgeons looking for a job. Below are interview tips from Helen Gammons. She has been a physician recruiter for 15 years, and when spoken to, said the most overlooked thing physicians do is not prepare for the interview. Below are her tips before going to interview for a position. The goal of the interview is to not only for the hiring entity to find a good fit, but for the physician to make sure they are a good fit for the position.

Interview Tips

- Do your homework—Go online and research the community and hospital so you will be familiar with it.
- Prepare a list of questions you want to ask.
- Once you receive the interview agenda also go online and research each individual you are scheduled to meet so that you will know a little bit about them when you meet with them. (You may have some common training, etc.)
- Be Professional. You do not have a second chance to make a first impression. We recommend that you wear a conservative suit, and have a neat and well-groomed appearance. Make sure that your clothing is clean, pressed, and presentable. Try to develop a rapport and relate with the interviewer. Always maintain eye contact and positive body language. Do not interrupt the interviewer and listen to them very closely. Always address whomever is interviewing you as Dr./Mr./Mrs. unless they tell you otherwise.

- Arrive a few minutes early.
- Maintain eye contact and show interest in everyone involved in the interview.
- DO NOT discuss salary. It's important to remember that you should never ask about salary during your first interview. If asked what kind of offer you are looking for, your response should be, "I will consider your strongest offer." This will prevent you from giving a figure that is too high or too low, which could take you out of the running because they can't afford you—or generate an offer less than desired. If and when they offer you the position, you can negotiate the offer and discuss your salary.
- DO NOT have more than one alcoholic drink at any meal or event with a potential employer.
- DO NOT take your spouse or significant other to you to the actual interview itself—this is only for the physician. The spouse or significant other is usually invited to come to the city to see it when you interview, but do not take that as an invitation to bring him/her with you when you meet everyone at the hospital or clinic on the actual interview day.
- Show equal respect to all you meet. (The receptionist is just as important as the Hospital CEO and in fact they will frequently ask the receptionist for his/her opinion of you).
- Follow up with a thank-you note to each interviewer. Even though it is common to just send an e-mail to thank someone, that is fine to do, but the hand written note will set you aside from others.
- Close the deal. Your goal in any interview is to get an offer. If you like what you see, don't leave the interview without letting the interviewer know you are really interested in the position.

Questions to Ask: (In No Particular Order).

- What is the call schedule?
- How many other physicians in the community will call be shared with them?

- How many calls and admissions do you handle on a typical call night or weekend?
- What is anticipated # of surgeries per month? (if you are a surgeon) or What is anticipated # of patients seen per day?
- DO NOT ask "How many patients do I need to see each day." A more appropriate question would be "What is the targeted # of patients that you would like a physician to see per day?" OR "How many patients per day do the physicians in the group typically see?"
- When you start practicing, do you receive feedback or education on billing and coding?
- How is productivity measured?
- If a surgeon, Is there block scheduling for surgery in the OR?
- If a surgeon, Do you use MD or CRNA Anesthesia or a combination of both?
- Do physicians hire and fire their own staff or does the hospital do that for you?
- Is there an office manager for the clinic or is the office manager in a centralized location?
- As the interview goes along—you will likely recognize some additional questions that you want to ask.

Behavior-based interviews have become popular recently, replacing loosely structured, traditional interviews. This type of interview allows employers to ask candidates questions about how they have handled previous situations, in an effort to predict future behavior. Behavioral interviewing is used to assist employers in finding a good match, lower turnover rates, and increase job satisfaction and performance. Behavioral interviewing focuses on asking about a situation in the past, the action taken to address the situation, and the outcome.

Tips for Preparing for an Interview

Be prepared. Questions will be based on your past experience. Therefore, have specific examples and situations prepared to share. If this job will be based on seeing patients, be prepared to answer questions such as, "Tell me about a time when you encountered a difficult patient who was unhappy with his or her service."

Beware of questions that ask for your mistakes or personal failings. Don't answer them in a way that will make the employer doubt your abilities. You can discuss something that was difficult, but end on a positive note by relating how you managed it.

Allow time to think of an appropriate answer, even if it requires a few moments of silence.

Answer each question concisely, with one example. Let interviewers ask if they want elaboration or another example.

Rehearse answers to potential questions ahead of time.

Here Are Some Examples of Interview Questions Using the Behavioral Interviewing Model

Tell me about a project or an idea that was successful mostly because of your efforts.

Think of a time when you had to make an important decision without enough information. Explain your decision-making process.

Tell me about a time when you encountered a difficult patient who was unhappy with his or her service.

Tell me about a time when something unexpected happened that changed the way you planned your day.

Tell me about a situation in which you had to overcome or manage an obstacle to accomplish your objectives.

Give me an example of a situation in which you found a new or improved way of doing something significant.

References

1. United States Department of Labor. Occupational outlook handout, 2008–2009 edition. https://www.bls.gov.
2. Primary Care. The Physician Recruiter. 2007;15(3):2–4.

3. Association of Women Surgeons. Finding and keeping your job as a surgeon: maximizing success. https://www.womensurgeons.org/wp-content/uploads/2015/03/Finding-and-Keeping-Your-Job-as-a-Surgeon-FINAL.pdf.

4. American College of Surgeons. Dimension 1: types of hospital/institution environments. Surgeons as institutional employees: a strategic look at the dimensions of surgeons as employees of hospitals. https://www.facs.org/~/media/files/advocacy/pubs/employed%20surgeon%20primer.ashx.

5. Weiss GG. Finding a job—Step 2: start looking. Medical Economics. Nov 2004, p. 14.

6. Schaefer CJ. The interview. Life after residency: a guide for the new physician and surgeon. https://www.facs.org/education/resources/rap/life-after-residency-a-guide-for-the-new-physician-and-surgeon.

7. Berra Y, Kaplan D. You can observe a lot by watching: what I've learned about teamwork from the Yankees and life. Hoboken: Wiley; 2008.

Chapter 2
Choosing the Right Job—How to Find the Right Fit, What Should I Look For?

Prashant Sinha

The experience of choosing a job as a surgeon is incomprehensibly complex. There are an increasing number of post-residency fellowships, an increasing demand for jobs with an expected 20% growth between 2012–2022, changing competency requirements, and increasing marketplace competition. The era of one job for a lifetime is gone, over 50% of physicians change jobs within the first 2 years [1], and practice patterns are rapidly changing. It is this incredible diversity that makes practicing surgery today, and for the foreseeable decades, more variable but also more personalized than ever before. What this means for your first or next job is that the more you look, the closer you get to ideal. A good job should find a match with an individual that sets realistic constraints and prioritizes their expectations with honesty. This chapter on choice should appeal to a diverse group of job seekers, and I will strive to provide tools to inform that choice as much as possible.

As background, I have lived my adult life in the US Northeast, not straying very far or for very long. My training and practice is and has been predominantly in academic

P. Sinha, M.D., F.A.C.S. (✉)
NYU Langone Medical Center,
530 First Ave, Suite 6C, New York, NY 10016, USA
e-mail: prashant.sinha@nyumc.org

© Springer International Publishing AG 2017
D.B. Renton et al. (eds.), *The SAGES Manual Transitioning to Practice*, DOI 10.1007/978-3-319-51397-3_2

medical centers, but I have deviated out of academia for a community practice, and I have practiced in fields outside of clinical medicine including finance, web development, and medical device development and have enjoyed every bit of it. I am not advocating for my particular choices though, as they reflect only my interests; choices should never be imposed on you when job seeking.

I presume that as job seekers, you will have chosen a specialty or focus in surgery that suits you well. Specific specialties will provide constraints of their own, particularly when a field requires regionalized referrals to a large medical center—transplant, surgical oncology, endocrine, and pediatric surgery for example. Beyond specialty, life circumstances will place particular constraints on choice, and it is very important to respect those constraints rather than ignore them. A prominent transplant surgeon told me that he started his job based on geography, and has never regretted it. It allowed him family stability and family support while he began his career, and subsequently allowed him to loosen geographic constraints when his family's needs changed. He changed jobs (and geography) twice since, each change fulfilling a specific career goal. Prioritize life constraints before choosing a job. Salary, predictability of hours, benefits, research, teaching, community or regional presence, commute, growth opportunity, and opportunities in unrelated or tangential fields; these are all different considerations among many more that can shape your future career or careers.

Salary is only one driver of choice, but one that is highly variable and highly subjective. Once a threshold is crossed, the value of salary may be secondary to other constraints. Most people will understand the drivers of and range of salary as they start their search within a given specialty and geography. As a general statement however, the Department of Labor and Statistic reports that the median general surgeon pay is $367,885 in 2015. There are significant variations depending on fellowship training, geography, and years of experience. The first year of practice in any setting is expected to generate a loss on the professional side. Most every entity, faculty practice, private practice group, and hospital employment, has a mechanism to manage this loss. Hospitals, for example, offset the employment overhead through new inpatient admissions, by pooling overhead costs with other surgeons, and by providing income guarantees to allow time for practice building. It is often for this reason that many contracts include a 1–3-year term for renewal allowing a mechanism to assess practice building and to manage the risks of a poorly performing surgeon. If income concerns are a top priority, choosing to practice in a large medical center will usually provide the most clinical volume stability with the least financial risk. Large medical centers recognize this and can afford to reduce salary commensurate with their stability and reputation. They count on longevity, productivity, and other factors like outcomes and academic contribution as metrics to increase salary. Surgeons that choose to diversify their practices can benefit from increased income and not always with significant increase in risk. Diversification may include combining high volume ambulatory procedures with more complex inpatient procedures. Alternative income strategies could also include investment into physician owned practices, or ambulatory care centers when allowed by law. Physicians that add administrative job duties within a hospital or large group practice have diversified their talents and income stream. Low-level administrative duties do not add income, but with progressive experience or targeted management training, physician leaders within a hospital or healthcare network are highly valued and can be compensated accordingly. Some private practice surgeons have used their creativity and entrepreneurship exceedingly well to add revenue. I personally know a few business-minded private practice surgeons that concurrently pursue medical device development while maintaining a hospital affiliation for referrals and continue to pursue scholarly activity through their professional society. Some have invested time and money in hobbies or fields entirely outside of medicine. Maintaining an efficient clinical practice can provide a solid financial base for almost anything, particularly when all aspects of the finances and clinical volume can be controlled as in private practice.

The next several sections will discuss the various venues for practicing surgeons, private practice, academic medicine, institutional medicine, and community hospital medicine. This will be followed by a concluding section summarizing the various aspects of these different types of practices and the types of personalities that are drawn to those types of practice.

Private Practice

It is still possible to have a successful private practice, even as a solo practitioner, but it is important to have a full understanding of what it entails. The private practitioner still exists in surgery in many parts of the country both urban and rural, although the overall trend has been toward employed positions. The pressures that have driven practitioners away from a solo practice into group or hospital owned practices are significant, mostly poor growth in reimbursement relative to office costs. A new requirement to switch to electronic medical records systems has unfortunately added to overhead costs. And, with overall payments decreasing relative to inflation, workloads have increased causing surgeon fatigue. However, the satisfaction of managing all aspects of a private practice can be very gratifying due to practice efficiency, capturing more of the gross income and actively control workload. The net income difference in private versus employed group employment has decreased though, and the ability to capture patient market share can be harder with managed care contracts, while benefits such as personal healthcare costs have increased. A decision to enter a private practice should weigh these issues particularly when an arrangement is being made to work at a hospital or ambulatory clinic. It will be important to understand how surgeons currently work at the facility that will support your surgical procedures, and also to understand how a hospital would view your entry into the market. You should understand whether your entry creates competition primarily or whether your entry comes with added skills that are not currently or readily available. There is a trend toward hospital acquisition of physician practices, particularly mature ones that serve patients that may choose between several hospitals. Hospitals make money with inpatient stays and referrals to inpatient services or ancillary services that are hospital owned. If possible, learn about any recent physician practice acquisitions before choosing to enter the market independently.

Three of my friends have nevertheless chosen the private practice route, and each of these has taken slightly different routes. The first, a plastic surgeon, freshly out of fellowship, currently practices in three locations—a rented office time-share in a cosmetic practice of an acquaintance, an ambulatory surgery center, and its affiliate hospital. He has chosen to define the scope of his practice to 10% cosmetic surgery with a well-established group as a contractor, and the remainder as reconstructive work focused primarily on breast oncology within a tertiary medical center with a cancer center and an affiliated ambulatory surgery center. His wife has become the business manager, and they have a wonderful work–life balance even if work is ever present in the background; that balance comes from the freedom of controlling their own workload. They have some risk as a solo practice, but these have been mitigated by having multiple relatively independent sources of revenue, and professional friendships that have allowed for mutually beneficial cross-coverage of patients. As time passes, his value in his community and his preferred hospital has continually increased leaving him with various opportunities—offers for practice buyout, transition to hospital employment, and requests for additional services. Next, an orthopedic hand surgeon chose to leave an academic practice where he was also a fellowship program director in order to build a better practice than the medical center provided, and one that clearly had need in the community. The process of starting the practice took a year of planning including a research phase, wind-down phase at the medical center, and a transition into practice phase. He hired a new fellow that he had personally trained, rented space in a building owned by an existing orthopedic practice with minimal clinical overlap, and is using a free EMR to keep overhead costs down. The loss of significant income as he transitions his practice has been mitigated by having had 15 years of local community presence and savings behind him and a family willing to ride out the change with him. Before he announced his intent to leave the medical center, his practice was ready to start business in case his leaving did not proceed well; it worked out well with an agreeable transition period. His long-term plan is to grow the practice into a multisite facility as a route to his own retirement and as a lasting legacy to the community in which he has practiced. The third example, a bariatric surgeon, had joined a stable general surgery practice out of fellowship and used it to build a successful bariatric practice—this surgeon was also his senior partner's prior resident. When the senior partner retired, he had to decide on selling or staying. Having had a good trajectory and an office staff already accustomed to the increased overhead in managing a high volume bariatric clinic practice, this surgeon hired a newly graduated fellow and a physician assistant. At the same time he completed a successful negotiation with a competing nearby hospital willing to help provide growth through larger and better facilities, a new referral pathway that would allow practice growth, and a 3-year proposal for practice purchase. This savvy surgeon understood his market value to a competitor hospital and allowed himself to be "bought" by his competitor as the market dynamics changed. He and his new hospital gained as his former affiliate lost. Local laws can also dramatically affect local market conditions, and these are particularly important to pay attention to. For my three friends above, the longest in private practice had an ambulatory procedure suite within his office, but the other two could not build office or ambulatory procedure suites due to increased regulatory oversight over their creation and maintenance.

If starting a private practice is daunting or a finding a partner is difficult, then the benefits of private practice can also be had through joining a solo or small group practice. Any more than three practitioners usually becomes a more complex organization requiring a management tier and likely a senior/junior partner structure; the partner or managing tier is typically a time-tenured or high volume member that collects a higher salary and/or has an equity stake in the practice. In most established private practice settings, there should be a strong pre-existing relationship to a hospital and or ambulatory surgery facility. Similarly, there should be strong ties to referring physicians and these relationships must be respected and maintained in the manner set by the practice. Similarly privileges in the operating suites may imply negotiated on call coverage that is either accounted for in the private practice or may be an additional requirement. Joining a private practice is very much akin to joining a family; much can be learned by spending a day or more at the practice to watch how it conducts its business. It is vital to understand whether you will be adding growth or replacing a member, and to the extent possible to understand the business rationale for hiring an additional member. Relative to joining a faculty practice in an academic medical center, there is much greater transparency in understanding your own value and contribution to a small private practice group. A private practice group is also more sensitive to variations in the local market, and requires a particularly good working relationship with your peers as the risks are shared. A smart private practice group should help new hires with clinical and networking support early to reduce potential risks early in the relationship.

Whether you choose to start your own private practice by taking call in a hospital and building a referral base, or join a small private practice, make sure you have a good grasp of what it takes to manage a business. Recognize that it can take a good year of planning to put in place an office space, EMR, contracts with insurers, credentialing at hospitals or ambulatory surgery centers, and establishing a relationship with referring physicians. A good lawyer or firm with experience in contracts for private physician practices is worth the seemingly exorbitant cost.

The choice to start or join a private practice requires a detailed understanding of running a business, managing staff, negotiating contracts, managing cash flow, and local market dynamics. It provides for professional independence, centers around patient care, and allows the practice to cater to a particular referral base or patient populace. Long-term patient relationships are formed, and strong professional relationships with referring physicians are required. It therefore tends to attract those with strong business management skills and a focus on patient care. For those unwilling to put any portion of their income at risk, those that foresee a potential job change for their spouse or partner, and those that need the stability of a large institution or benefits that come with institutional backing, private practice is not the right fit. If teaching and research are important, this is not the environment to find those opportunities apart from some teaching as a part of hospital privileging requirements or as part of a professional society.

Academic Medicine

Our medical education curriculum has been structured to provide a basis for both clinical medicine and research, and as such prestige for medical schools and universities comes from a hybrid of clinical reputation and research funding and often colors our perception of our own future in medicine. Few surgeons are uniquely gifted to conduct both basic science and clinical medicine; however, many do partner with basic scientists and statisticians to collaboratively conduct translational and outcomes research in a wide variety of fields. Consider that NIH funding as of early 2000 to medicine departments contributed about 28% of NIH awards to a medical school and correlated strongly with the NIH rank for that school while only 4.8% of NIH grants went to surgical

departments of which general surgery took the largest share
[2]. Further consider that more recently in the decade ending
in 2013, surgical NIH funding decreased 19% with a propor-
tional tripling in outcomes research funding [3] and you
understand what a rarefied opportunity Academic Surgery is.
For those individuals trained in this environment, jobs are
highly competitive, geographically sparse and have pressures
exemplified by the phrase "triple threat"—excellence in
teaching, research, and clinical medicine. The barriers to entry
for those trained outside of this environment are much
higher. Fortunately, any motivated young surgeon that makes
their way into academia is well equipped to conduct clinical
and outcomes research with relatively little training in comparison to bench and translational research. The other unspo-
ken truth is that clinical surgery has a highly valuable
contribution to the bottom line in any hospital including the
most prestigious of academic medical centers. A productive
clinician may survive in an academic environment without
significant academic contributions through excellent outcomes and a regional reputation that draws referrals.
Conversely, a surgeon that is either not clinically productive
or fails to provide the latest advances in surgical care does
not have longevity.

   There are not many headhunters with postings for jobs in
academia. Many of these positions are filled through word-
of-mouth, often through a network of fellowships, and
through the social networks of mentors and leaders in academia. Fellowships often provide a path to the "academic
circuit" of publications, national meetings, posters, podium
presentations, book chapters, committees, and the like. While
this path is not necessarily an equal opportunity endeavor, it
does select individuals that can thrive in academia. Simply
having a track-record of excellent teaching is not sufficient;
however, the ability to combine a reputation as an educator
with another pillar of academia is highly desired and is a hall-
mark of those that have patience and well-developed cogni-
tive skills needed to lead cutting edge clinical care. Taking
time to develop a highly technical skill such as laparoscopic

liver surgery requires an investment of time and likely money (or personal debt) and may be a path into academic medicine, but again requires time spent on the national or international meeting circuit, and must be combined with publications and other scholarly activities. A technical skill can be highly desirable but may also become a commodity with time, such as laparoscopy and bariatric surgery. Furthermore, a highly technical skill may require casting a wide net geographically to find a regional medical center to support the procedure and attract patients.

Publish and get on the circuit; those two activities will put you on the roadmap and will focus your thinking. At the same time, accept the constraints of regionalized medicine. Have a realistic discussion with your family and partner, decide on what priority to give geographic constraints if any, and carve out a finite timeline for developing a reputation—don't let the pursuit of entering academic medicine last more than a typical fellowship timeframe of 1–3 years. That timeframe should also result in scholarly activity presented in meetings. Remember that with the constraints of academic medicine, your particular talents should fit in well with a few centers that either have a reputation in your interests or have committed to developing that interest. Mentorship is very important—researchers with a proven track-record during protected time in residency will often gain active guidance in finding an academic job or be recruited. Mentorship should be actively sought as a trainee or junior attending builds their interests and reputation. Mentors help guide development and greatly aid in finding and choosing a job in academia. For most others that are interviewing, it is important to spend time independently researching an institution as much as possible in advance, and to obtain information from fellows, residents, and any others. To the extent it matters, it will be valuable to understand what expectations are placed in terms of teaching commitments, publishing, clinical volume and protected time, and the particular cultural quirks. An academic job should also support several areas of interest for a given applicant, but will also require various amounts of clinical work. Questions should be focused on the tools needed to facilitate areas of academic interest and research—grant writing resources, core facility support for statistics, clinical trials, tissue banking, etc. If a commitment is made by the medical center to support a new procedure or new research techniques, particularly if capital equipment and labor resources are needed, then these should be included in the hiring contract and carefully reviewed. These are not common scenarios for junior surgical attendings but may arise when an established and talented individual is interviewing or recruited from one academic center to another, or from a highly regarded nonacademic institution into academia.

A job in academia is highly rewarding to those individuals that strive for that "triple threat" of patient care, teaching, and research. This environment is at the forefront of scientific breakthroughs and innovative approaches to care. It attracts a diverse group of patients and with them a diverse and at times challenging set of diseases and disorders, fulfilling to a surgeon interested in a broad exposure. With that type of clinical exposure, all types of research including clinical outcomes, innovative therapies, and systems of care and quality become productive and meaningful endeavors.

Institutional Practice

There is a world of opportunity to those academic-minded individuals that have not found a job at their preferred academic medical center, or that are primarily concerned with cutting edge patient care at a large hospital. These large institutional hospitals without associated medical schools are regional magnet hospitals that are known for advanced therapies and excellent patient outcomes, and even research. These institutions have typically developed clinical expertise in a few areas that may be nationally or even internationally known, have built operational excellence, and may even bring in substantial research funding. Recently, some institutions have become large conglomerates seeking to control both tertiary care centers and ambulatory care centers and physician practices across a given region. This network building serves to capture more patients within the network and create bargaining power with insurers, and hopefully improve care delivery (think Kaiser Permanente). Similar to academic medical centers, there is a large hospital affiliated practice with a well-established business unit that provides billing and administrative support, malpractice, and benefits. With a stronger focus on clinical medicine, and more of a business-minded focus, there may be less room for negotiation of salary, less influence of academic contributions to your value, but better benefit packages, more clinical flexibility, and improved call coverage. These institutions proudly market their accomplishments, and broadly publish their long-term goals and vision; it will be very important to think about your own alignment with those stated goals. Institutions competing in a region may employ surgeons to help with expansion when certain competencies (i.e., robotic liver surgery) are needed to compete with other institutions, or to develop a cutting edge therapy, or to fill a vacancy in a well-developed practice.

The interviews for jobs in these types of institutions are more likely to have been posted or have been sent to a recruiter to find particular types of candidates. A job may have the hybrid feel of a private practice job and an academic medical center. Important questions include the clinical productivity requirements, single versus multisite practice locations, and the frequency of rotating through those sites. Salary and increases in salary may or may not be negotiable, but can be significantly better than an academic medical center depending on the region. Generous fringe benefits can at times supplant a salary raise, while operational excellence makes focusing on clinical care easy in this type of setting. Compared to a private practice, however there are likely more restrictions on the scope of practice, and in how a practice can be developed. Having management skills can be leveraged within these institutions as their complex structure depends on good leadership. Similar to private practice, it is advisable to understand your own worth to the institutions goals and to plan your personal growth with the institutional vision. If a choice has to be made between an academic medical center and a nonacademic institution, benefits and resources that are available for clinical or research work are useful to compare and contrast. The culture of an institution is often set in the preceding decade, but it is very important to ask specifically about culture, shared values, and areas of change. The broader market in healthcare can subtly or dramatically force both academic and institutional centers to change the way they support clinicians and researchers. Major recent trends include increasing scrutiny in the granting and the maintenance of tenure in academia, in broadening racial diversity in the faculty, and in improving access to family support for an increasingly female workforce and in bending the cost curve. I myself have become increasingly engaged in the discipline of value-based medicine as an academic area of development alongside acute care outcomes, and advanced endoscopy. Heavy financial pressures on even very strong medical centers have placed increasing pressure on the individual clinician to become more cost conscious. Actively assessing what is on the mind of your future institution will give you a glimpse of your future within it.

In summary, institutional medical centers provide the closest clinical comparison to academic medical centers and have a central motivation on providing high volume, high quality and cutting edge clinical care. They care as much about their brand as an academic center, and may even have expertise in conducting research to rival the best academic medical centers. Compared to private practice, there is less schedule or practice flexibility, but a greater number of fringe and healthcare and retirement benefits. Salary as a private practitioner versus employee may or may not be competitive depending on the dominance of the institution on the overall local market; it may be better to join a dominant institution than to fight for market share.

Hospitals

Many hospitals do not fit into the model of institutional or academic medical center, but serve as the central focus of most surgeons. Hospitals can be fairly general or can be focused on specialties such as a cancer-focused hospital, a heart and vascular hospital, or hospital that has an associated ambulatory surgery center disease-focused on breast oncology. A disease or specialty-focused hospital can be a very rewarding place to work owing to operational efficiency. A community hospital may provide financial stability compared with private practice, while supporting lower volumes or lower complexity cases compared with a more urban setting. Choosing a hospital to work in should reflect your life priorities and how you conduct business at the hospital depends on your mode of employment; do you thrive with productivity targets, or would you rather work at your own pace. The preceding sections may already give a good flavor of what to expect in terms of employment by a hospital. This section will review many of the points made already and help the reader evaluate employment within a hospital. There are various models of employment that can be drawn up. There are a few basic parts that are combined in various ways. I will use my own experience as illustration.

I decided for various reasons to find a job within commuting distance for a year while I decided on my long-term goals. I found a job posting by a placement agency and very quickly found myself in a small community working in their local 100-bed hospital with five operating rooms and with a partner that was hired just before me. Before I moved back to an academic medical center, I knew that I would miss the more relaxed pace of performing community surgery as a hospital-employed surgeon, and I learned about my individual value to the hospital as a surgeon. Finally, more important than all of the benefits and salary models to be discussed below, the key to a successful practice is to have peers that are trustworthy and easy to work with.

I received a base salary for 2 years to allow for practice building. At the time, it was a significantly higher amount by almost 50% than the salary being offered by an academic medical center. After the 2 years, my compensation would switch to a base salary plus work-based compensation. The base would change based on the prior years income and additional payments would come from RVUs. Work Relative Value Units (wRVUs) are a unit of measure that is used to calculate physician payment for a specific procedure performed. RVU models are commonplace and take into account the complexity of the cases performed. A surgeon may decide to pick a volume/complexity mix that works well. A more complex case requires more work and generates more RVUs and inpatient management time while an ambulatory setting may allow easier, high volume low RVU cases. The number of RVUs is ultimately multiplied by a base payment that accounts for regional cost of living, your specialty, and perhaps additional amounts to reflect productivity. Because the formulas can be confusing, I asked that quarterly reports of my RVU work be provided along with the associated income as if I were on that model, while I developed my practice. The models are for the most part fair and are calculated by various agencies to help hospitals recruit and retain physicians. Some RVU models do not use a base level of salary but tiers to reflect different amounts of work; at the first tier, the RVU payment multiplier is lowest, rising for the next tier(s). Other payment models can use billing or collections and sometimes employers will pool those payments for a group of physicians to allow for practice variations and differences in productivity. If your salary is based on billing or collections, and you change jobs, there may be a large amount of money that will be pending (accounts receivable) as you wind down and it is best to discuss how and to whom this amount will be distributed once you leave and the money arrives. RVU models can be advantageous in some settings with a poorly insured patient populace as the wRVU for a surgeon does not depend on how much is actually collected.

Benefits should be available including healthcare, provisions for retirement contributions or even an employer match, malpractice coverage, CME funds or meeting and travel funds. New equipment purchases for specialty procedures, office space, physician extender support, discounted disability, and life insurance can also be part of a benefits package. Generally speaking, the larger the hospital the better the benefits, and while my hospital provided a very nice office space and excellent staff, there was little in the way of CME funds and no budget for physician extenders.

Loan repayments are not common but exist in underserved or critical access hospitals, and through the uniformed services as well as eight governmental agencies: National Institutes of Health; Food and Drug Administration; Centers for Disease Control; Alcohol, Drug Abuse, and Mental Health Administration; Health Resources and Services Administration; Agency for Health Care Policy and Research; Agency for Toxic Substances and Disease Registry; and Indian Health Service. For the eight governmental agencies, most will not support clinical surgery but may support related research, with the exception of the Indian Health Service. I know of surgeons in the Indian Health Service and in the Army and Navy; each of them has had challenging but gratifying experiences and careers. Both military and nonmilitary services are run with specific requirements and promotions as well as duty obligations. These will be discussed in a later chapter. Major additional benefits beyond loan repayment include exposure to global health and the ability to directly contribute to underserved populations, paid leave, travel benefits, and retirement benefits. Outside of these special government agencies, it may be worthwhile to ask about loan repayment from a prospective hospital employer in an underserved or rural area.

Malpractice coverage comes in two flavors, occurrence based and claims made. Private practice physicians will need to purchase this independently, but this is important to understand for any surgeon, particularly if there is any job or location change. Occurrence-based coverage allows you to change jobs or location and still be covered for the care delivered before the change. Claims-made coverage requires the purchase of a "tail" policy to allow coverage for any claims that arise after you leave. The individual surgeon may pay for this; however, it is common to negotiate this coverage with either the previous employer or the new employer.

Summary

Ultimately, there are more choices and more benefits available to surgeons today than there has been in the past. While payments have decreased and have become bundled, and administrative burdens have increased, a surgical career remains highly gratifying, and can be tailored to suit an individuals needs. There is no perfect job, and compromise is key while understanding the various modes of employment. I again emphasize that priorities should be given to personal needs, whether that is a salary goal, work–life balance, research, teaching, high complexity, low complexity, geography, service, or loan repayment. Some of the best advice comes from peer networking and mentors whether formal or informal, and meetings at professional societies. Some of the best job opportunities come from the same. Many of the concerns in choosing a job in various environments are listed here and hopefully each describes the atmosphere of that environment well. Choose based on your own research and ask important questions of your future employer and future peers. Remember that your needs may change or evolve over time, and in no way should you feel tied to one job for life. Finally, any job that you take will benefit from your own hard work, keeping in mind that the first several years require patience and extra dedication so that your expectations come to fruition.

References

1. United States Department of Labor. Occupational Outlook Handbook, 2008–09 Edition. Available at www.bls.gov (accessed October 5, 2016).
2. Ozomaro U et al. How important is the contribution of surgical specialties to a medical school's NIH funding? J Surg Res. 2007;141(1):16–21.
3. Hu Y et al. Recent trends in National Institutes of Health funding for surgery: 2003 to 2013. Am J Surg. 2015;209(6):1083–9.

Chapter 3
Contract Negotiations: Pitfalls and Traps When Reviewing Your Contract

Charles Paget and Allison Farris

Introduction

The most important thing to recognize is that signing a contract is a process of negotiation. You have interviewed, and the practice or hospital wishing to hire you makes a contract offer. Now the fun begins. A contract can elucidate a lot about the job, the expectations, and the dark secrets the potential employer may not want you to know. It should also lay out the conditions of employment in years to come and how one becomes a partner. Even if you expect that this is only an initial contract and new one will be offered after the first years of practice, it is vitally important to get the initial contract right.

C. Paget, B.S., M.D. (✉)
Department of Surgery, Carilion Clinic Virginia Tech
School of Medicine, 1906 Bellview Avenue, Medical Education
Building, Room 302, Roanoke, VA 24014, USA
e-mail: cjpaget@carilionclinic.org

A. Farris, M.D.
Department of Surgery, Carilion Health System,
Roanoke, VA, USA
e-mail: arfarris@carilionclinic.org

© Springer International Publishing AG 2017   33
D.B. Renton et al. (eds.), *The SAGES Manual Transitioning
to Practice*, DOI 10.1007/978-3-319-51397-3_3

Basics

Much of contractual text is about money, and most people focus on guaranteed salary and potential income. The well-advised negotiator understands that the amount of money is less important than other issues. If you are not happy and successful in your practice, you are not likely to stay. If you and your family are not happy living in this new location, it does not matter how much you are paid. Finally, if you feel you have been treated unfairly, even if this is subjective and you are paid well, you will not stay. A clear understanding of expectations, both those stated explicitly in your contract and those not clearly stated, contributes more to this sense of fairness than anything else might. The most important factor in negotiating a satisfying contract is preserving the sense that you are valued as a person and a surgeon, and decreasing surprises to come.

Non-compete clauses are inserted to prevent a physician from being supported by a private practice or hospital for the first several years, only to leave for independent practice or a place in a competing group. The employer has invested money in you as a new employee and wants protection for this investment. If you are going to a small town with a single hospital or single private practice, this clause is largely unimportant, as if you do not like the situation you are more likely to leave town. If you intend to stay in the area, these clauses increase in importance. Non-compete clauses usually specify a geographic area (i.e., a 20 mile circle from the primary office) and a time limit (such as 1–2 years). The feasibility of enforcing these varies by state. Often there is buyout clause (1 year salary, their investment) or ways of negotiating out of this. If the hospital thinks a provider will continue to bring business to them, they may allow an employee leaving with proper stipulations.

There are several methods for moving from employee to partner in a private surgery practice. Some practices require a buy-in after a certain period of being an employee (usually 1–2 years). Other groups may require you to work for a certain period of time (maybe 4–5 years) until you are made a partner. Much of this depends upon your salary guarantee. If you are paid near market average for a general surgeon at the outset, the corporation that is employing you will lose money on you in the first several years. The expectation is that after an appropriate learning curve and ramping up of your practice, the income you bring in will offset this loss. This would suggest that in years 3–5 you are paid less than you are actually earning to offset the loss from the first few years. All of these methods are fair in the long run under the right circumstances.

"Buy-in" refers to when a new partner is required to put forth a certain sum of money to purchase shares in the corporation that is the practice. Typically a "buy-in" is for an equal share in the practice, i.e., for a group with four partners the buy-in would convey one quarter of all assets. Note this includes only hard assets such as building cost, computers, and equipment. Many practices separate the building ownership from the rest of these assets and the practice rents the space, even if several partners own the building. Often the hard assets are less than $100,000 in a small practice, so the buy-in is not that onerous. Those who are buying into a practice should make sure the buy-in (or stock in the corporation) is recoverable if you leave the practice, and understand how these assets may be recovered.

Signing Bonuses and Other Ways to Sweeten the Deal

Several other incentives can be added to a contract to sweeten the deal. These often depend on the difficulty of recruiting to the position and the expected income you can generate for the practice. The first of these is a signing bonus that can be paid well prior to starting the job. If you have family expenses and little savings upon graduation, a signing bonus can help a lot. Moving expenses are often negotiated into a contract deal as well. Medical school loan forgiveness is available in some rural areas and especially in critical access hospitals. These can be substantial and worth losing money on other salary if your loan debt is sizeable. Money for continuing education, disability insurance, and health insurance are all part of the contract in many cases, especially when working for a hospital or large multispecialty group. Each of these is a separate but related part of the negotiation. The employer may be willing to give you a larger signing bonus but decrease the salary guarantee, effectively front loading your yearly salary. You may not get everything you ask for, but you cannot know until you ask. Finally, retirement plans and contributions to a 401K (private practice and for-profit corporations) or 403B (not for profit corporations) are important, and these need to be considered when evaluating the employment offer. In a private practice group, you typically finance your own 401K, essentially trading take-home pay for investment as pretax income in your retirement plan. Within a larger corporation, part of retirement usually comes out of your salary, as above, and is matched by the corporation.

Models of Reimbursement

You need to understand the concept of risk and reward in terms of salary and bonus calculation. The more money you are guaranteed, the lower the ceiling for your top earning, and vice versa in a properly written contract. Some groups split earnings equally amongst the partners. The benefits of this model include decreasing competition among members of a group, but it only works if the same work ethic is shared amongst all the partners. The opposite extreme is a pure production model, or "eat what you kill," where each partner's earnings are directly garnered from his or her collections. This means any low pay or no pay patients, which are often those patients seen by the junior partner, produce significantly less reimbursement for time and effort expended. There are also a variety of very good hybrid models, consisting of a base salary plus some percentage (often 25–50%) derived from production. The measure that is used for determining production is important. Production measured on collections rather than billings tends to favor the established partners. Well-insured patients often seem to make it to the senior partner, while the uninsured are seen by the new partner. Many larger groups or hospital-owned practices base production on relative value units (RVUs) that are available across specialties and offer a measure of production that is not based on collections. In an RVU-based system, payer mix does not affect physician productivity numbers.

Payment for anyone in a surgical practice is based on the following concept: you bill a certain amount and collect a percentage (typically 30–50%) of that. Overhead costs (rent, employee salaries and benefits, and liability insurance) are subtracted from collections. The amount remaining is available to pay the physicians. In the older purely production model, physicians essentially worked for the first 3–4 months to pay the overhead for the year, then everything made beyond that was take-home pay. This meant a partner with 25% more collections might make twice the salary as each partner contributes an equal amount to overhead. Although this system seems to reward the more industrious, it actually tends to preserve the status quo. It also tends to produce competition between partners. As overhead began to creep up, and simultaneously collections decreased, the number of months worked to cover overhead stretched from 3–4 months to sometimes 6–9 months. However in the RVU model, the first and last RVU earn the same amount for the physician, with the larger corporation taking both the risk of falling short of the overhead and the benefit of surplus collections. RVU systems can be based purely on production, but are often hybrid systems where a base salary is given and any RVUs generated beyond a certain level are compensated on a dollar amount per RVU.

You are unlikely to change the model of reimbursement during your negotiation, but it is important to understand the various models and how they could affect you. The number of partners in your group, the number of surgeons in town, and the overall growth of medical care (or lack thereof) will affect *your* production, as a new surgeon, more than that of any established partners or practices.

Initial Contract Versus Long-Term Agreement

Some contracts are written to cover only the first few years of employment. If they do, you absolutely need to see a copy of permanent contract or partnership agreement. Also the initial contract needs to specify the pathway and expectations that lead to partnership. The expectations on a year by year basis need to be spelled out and a goal of the negotiation is to determine if these are realistic. Many contracts have a hefty guarantee for the first year but expect the new surgeon to be able to fully support themselves by the second or third year. As with many of the other parameters discussed, the more risk you assume financially, the more the financial upside should be in terms of possible bonus beyond base salary. If the position is as an employed surgeon, as is typical with a hospital or large healthcare employer, the contract may not change after the first year as you are not progressing towards partnership. These contracts will still have methods by which your salary grows over the years and you need to understand these methods.

Malpractice Insurance

Most contracts include the type of malpractice insurance offered and how it is paid. Malpractice insurance may be part of your overhead in a private practice group and is paid in pretax dollars as a business expense. As an employee of a hospital/health system, malpractice insurance is simply part of employment and may not be a line item expense. It is more important to know if the policy is a claims-made policy or occurrence-based policy. An occurrence-based policy is clearly preferable. An occurrence policy protects you from any covered incident that *occurs* during the policy period, regardless of when the claim is filed. Claims-made policies provide coverage for claims only when BOTH the alleged incident AND the resulting claim happen during the period the policy is in force. Claims-made policies provide coverage so long as the insured continues to pay premiums for the initial policy and any subsequent renewals. If you move your practice or retire with a claims-made policy, you are required to purchase "Tail Coverage" from the insurance company that covers any events that occurred during the insured period but were filed as claims after the policy ended. The longer you are in practice, the higher the cost of the tail coverage, and it is often several times the annual premium and can be greater than a year's salary. Occurrence policies are increasingly difficult to find, but the larger healthcare entities often self-insure and can offer these occurrence policies. One exception to tail coverage occurs when a practice decides to switch malpractice carriers. In this case, the new carrier usually covers any claims made under the new insured period for incidents that occurred during prior coverage, in addition to claims from incidents that occur during the new period. This makes switching insurance carriers based on competitive rates realistic.

Getting Out of a Contract

A significant percentage of new surgeons will spend only 2–3 years at their initial job, indicating a lack of fit or failed expectations. This works both ways as you may not have your contract renewed or you may not be offered partnership. The initial contract should spell out the period of time within which this decision is made. Many surgeons will also move for career advancement or new opportunities. Most contracts allow surgeons to walk away from their contract without penalty if they are leaving the area. However, you may be required to stay a nominal length of time (2–3 years) or pay back the signing bonus or salary guarantee. Salary guarantees are becoming the norm for at least the first year of practice, and most employers wish to protect this investment. It is important to know what amount of production (as measured by collections or RVUs) allows you to cover your salary. It is likely you will not cover the guaranteed salary in your first year of practice, so it is necessary to know what your obligations are in terms of paying this back if you choose to leave the practice. It is also important to know what occurs if you exceed production expectations. Leaving a contract but staying in the area is a more tricky proposition and the wording of the original non-compete clause becomes important. A surgeon in private practice who operates at a hospital brings about a half million dollars to that hospital annually in ancillary charges, radiology, operating room charges, and inpatient reimbursement. If you have chosen to leave the employment of the hospital, you may be able to negotiate your way out of the contract if you continue to operate and admit at that hospital. The hospital will continue to benefit even if you do not directly work for them. Alternately you or your new employer can buy out your contract from the previous employer, thus allowing you to remain in the same city. These all depend upon local needs, employment structure, and your willingness to compromise.

Considerations

A few points to consider if you are new surgery residency or fellowship graduate: you will not be nearly as efficient or fast in the operating room. You will need to learn a new system of clinic, hospital, and support staff and adapt them to your own needs. Typically you will be sent fewer and less healthy patients initially. If you have been in practice for a number of years, this change is less noticeable. Specialist bringing new talents to an area often becomes busier faster than generalists. That all being said, it likely will take you 3–5 years at least to get to a level of efficiency that allows you to earn that amount upon which most measures of average salary are based. Employers know this, and account for it when calculating salaries and bonuses. They also realize that everyone's work ethic and desire to produce varies a great deal. Understand that fair contracts are fair for both sides. Many surgeons would not want the contracts that come with the highest salary as that requires the highest production which can affect time with family and availability for teaching. It can also engender the feeling that your only purpose is production rather than why you got into medicine in the first place.

When reading an offer, consider if it is a modification of a contract a 1000 physicians have signed, or if it is one of the first the prospective employer has written. In the latter case, there is likely much more latitude for change. In the former, you probably have limited room for negotiation but the main negotiation point will be base salary. The negotiation often demonstrates the trustworthiness of your future employers and the factors important to them.

Finally, be aware that median incomes for surgeons vary widely based on a number of factors. One key driver of median salary is geographic area, but surgical specialty, population of the area, and healthcare needs can also have a great effect. More information on physician salaries can be found from a variety of sources including MedScape, and some research in this area can be very beneficial when evaluating offers.

As mentioned previously, many contracts include productivity measures based on RVUs as this gives a standard measure of production that is not influenced by payor mix, unlike either billings or collections. Compensation correlates directly with RVUs as indicated in Table 3.1. Compare the number of RVUs produced by surgeons earning in the 25th percentile to those earning in the 75th percentile. As expected, increased RVU productivity has a direct effect on compensation. Also remember this data presents total compensation including base salary, bonuses, and the value of all benefits for surgeons at a given percentile. It has been reported by the Medical Group Management Association (MGMA), an organization that collects data for larger organizations to see what competitors across the country are paying. The quoted numbers are for private practice, and a separate set of data is available

TABLE 3.1 General surgery RVU and average compensation by percentile[a]

	25th Percentile	Median	75th Percentile	90th Percentile
RVUs	4951	6750	8709	11,017
Compensation	$321,262	$395,456	$504,323	$645,687

[a]MGMA Data, 2015 report based on 2014 data. ©2015 MGMA. All rights reserved. Data Extracted from MGMA Datadrive

for academic practice. Although it illustrates the relationship between RVU production and compensation, there is no indication in this data of the amount of compensation derived from other sources. A section leader at a major institution may only be producing the median number of RVUs but is also paid for his administrative time so that his total salary is much higher than his production numbers would indicate. This may explain why data from MGMA shows much higher compensation than what is reported in the Medscape survey. Also, an institution may pay significantly more to certain subspecialists in order to keep a service available. As such MGMA data gives only a rough approximation of what is actually being paid. Understand that larger institutions have this data and use it to guide their salary structure. They also may demand other forms of work such as administrative or teaching time in addition to clinical production to justify these salaries.

Red Flags to Avoid

There are several red flags that should make you think twice before agreeing to a contract. One example is a partner's family member acting as office manager. Another example is if partners within the group are already distrustful of one another. In this situation you, as the new employee, are placed in the awkward position of negotiating between the established partners. Avoid any practice offer where there is not a clear need for another surgeon in town or in the group; a desire to increase the call pool is never a good reason to hire another surgeon unless there is also plenty of business to go around during the day. Finally, think carefully before being hired by a solo practitioner as his or her initial partner. If this is just prior to retirement, get a projected retirement date set in writing. For this arrangement to be succesful, a practice that was supporting one surgeon would have to increase its production by 75–100% at least in the short term. It is much easier to become the fifth surgeon in a group of four where the marginal increase is only 15–20%. A group or surgeon that is planning to hire a new partner should, in the short term, be willing to see their own production fall. If they have not realized this or are unwilling to give up some of their income for the benefit of having a new partner, they are not being realistic.

Let's conclude with some examples.

Example 1

You would be the fifth member of a private practice that recently saw retirement of their senior partner. The present four members are working to the point of exhaustion. They are in a mid-sized town with six other general surgeons in the area. The hospital is doing well and the area is growing in population. You are offered a generous first year salary but with bonus only if you exceed 9000 RVUs. In that case your bonus would consist of 25% of excess collections. Your salary is to hold steady for 5 years and then you become a partner.

Consider, is this contract fair or not fair? How busy do you expect to be?

Example 2

You would be joining a three surgeon group in a small town that has recently lost their junior partner. They are the only surgeon group in town. They offer you a low entry salary but with bonus if you exceed collections needed to pay your own overhead and salary. Overhead is split percentage wise by collections, i.e. the partner with highest collections pays the highest proportion of the overhead. The bonus is a direct dollar for dollar amount after coverage of your guaranteed salary and overhead.

Is this contract fair or not fair? Again, how busy do you expect to be?

Example 3

You would be joining a group of ten surgeons practicing as part of a large, multispecialty group owned by a hospital. You are offered a base salary which is near the average for the region. The contract states you are expected to generate 7000 RVUs the first year and will be paid extra for every RVU beyond the 7000 threshold. There is potential for a bonus that is dependent upon multiple factors that change from year to year based on the hospital's goals. Each year your base salary can be changed based on your production from the year before but will never decrease by more than 5% per year. Your base salary will mirror the RVU target so that as base salary goes up, the RVU target goes up. You inquire about the language of the contract and are told this is same contract offered to every physician employed by the hospital regardless of specialty with the only differences being base salary and the amount of expected administration time.

Fair or not fair? How busy will you be?

Example 4

You would be the first partner of a 50-year-old surgeon whose practice has been very successful and who has been pushed by the local hospital to recruit a partner to this smaller market. The five other surgeons in town are all in private practice. The hospital believes the volume is growing. They have capacity for growth and feel this will continue. You are offered a 1 year guarantee of $300,000 by the hospital.

You will split the overhead with your partner. Any collections of yours beyond overhead will go towards your salary with the hospital kicking in to make up any difference. Second year you are on pure production model and the hospital is no longer guaranteeing your salary.

Fair or not? How busy?

Example 1: Discussion

This group expects you to be busy out of the gate, and if you are not it will be your own fault. A 9000 RVU goal for the first year out of training is a mark you are unlikely to achieve. The group has offered you what they estimate you will average over 5 years. They should be willing to show you their average RVU production and one would expect them to be in the range of 10000 per year. If you fall far short of collecting what they are paying you for the first 2 years they may not renew your contract. The minimal bonus is a signal that they are taking a risk by paying a high salary guarantee. Overall, this offer indicates that they want a long-term partner and this is a good position.

Example 2: Discussion

This is a fair offer, but do not expect the group to help you to become busy right away as it is not in their best interest. Be skeptical as to why the junior partner left. He may have never been able to compete with the two older, more established surgeons. This is a contract that can be good if you are willing to stay a significant amount of time and establish yourself, so this needs to be a location in which you and your family can happily live long term. The economic health and growth of the area will be important factors in deciding to take this offer. It is very reasonable to ask to speak to the prior partner who has left, and one would expect the remaining senior partners to introduce you to him or her. This stipulation allows you to gauge your prospective partners' honesty and transparency.

Example 3: Discussion

This contract is fair. You have significant downside protection and the ability to increase your earnings. Your chief negotiating point would be the starting base salary. It is difficult to tell from the information provided how busy you may be, the relative number of surgeons (increasing or decreasing), any new talents you bring to the area, and the nature of your practice. A practice which is mostly electively scheduled operations takes longer to build than one in which you are scheduled to staff an inpatient service for a week at a time. The RVU estimate is realistic for the first year, and the contract has built in plans for re-evaluation on a yearly basis. This offer from a larger, multispecialty group likely has multiple non-salary benefits as well, so total compensation needs to be big part of the decision.

Example 4: Discussion

This is very risky contract after the first year. Increasing a single person practice to a two person partnership will require nearly doubling the production of the practice, which seems unlikely to happen. Secondly, the established surgeon has no incentive to help his new partner increase his or her business. It is impossible to tell how busy you will be. This contract needs a clearer statement of long-term plans and better contribution by the senior partner or hospital. This is a contract that may mean you are looking for a new job in two years, or it may work out well. You and your family's willingness to move if this does not work out is an important point to consider prior to accepting this offer.

Conclusion

When evaluating an employment contract there are many factors to contemplate. Every applicant must weigh his or her priorities when considering an employment offer. For example, some may wish to maximize earning potential early with the plan to move to another position after a few years. Others may be looking for a long-term fit with a larger portion of reimbursement contributed by retirement and other benefits. There is no correct answer for which factor matters most as it varies for each individual. Do be sure to be honest with yourself and your potential employers about what you are hoping to achieve through the negotiation. The input of your family can be invaluable, as they will be sharing this journey with you. Finally, though you are now armed with a basic knowledge of contractual jargon and the underlying meanings, it is always beneficial to have a trusted mentor review a contract prior to acceptance. With a firm understanding of what to expect and an idea of what your priorities are, plus a little guidance along the way, you are sure to find a satisfying contract that will fulfill your personal and professional goals.

Chapter 4
How Do I Get Paid: Medicare, Medicaid, Insurance, Billing Pearls

Charles Paget, Don J. Selzer, and Allison Farris

Introduction

However you are paid and whatever type of practice you join, you need to know how to bill to justify your salary. Whether you are in a large hospital-owned practice where reimbursement is based on RVUs or in private practice and paid out of accounts receivable, maximizing billing improves reimbursement and eventually your take-home pay. Many surgeons think billing is too complicated for them to bother learning and would rather send operative notes to their coders and hope for the best. But there are many good reasons why every surgeon needs to understand billing.

C. Paget, B.S., M.D. (✉)
Department of Surgery, Carilion Clinic Virginia Tech
School of Medicine, 1906 Bellview Avenue,
Medical Education Building, Room 302, Roanoke, VA 24014, USA
e-mail: cjpaget@carilionclinic.org

D.J. Selzer, M.D., M.S.
Division of General Surgery, Department of Surgery,
Indiana University School of Medicine

A. Farris, M.D.
Department of Surgery, Carilion Health System,
Roanoke, VA, USA
e-mail: arfarris@carilionclinic.org

© Springer International Publishing AG 2017
D.B. Renton et al. (eds.), *The SAGES Manual Transitioning to Practice*, DOI 10.1007/978-3-319-51397-3_4

49

You will always miss opportunities to be paid if you do not understand the rules. Imagine a professional football coach that did not know the ever changing NFL rules, and how difficult it would be for that coach to win. Taking this a step further, millions of fantasy football fans watch and know every rule of the NFL despite yearly changes. Surely, every surgeon is as capable as any of these fans; it is simply a matter of motivation. Understanding which words or descriptions identify an operation as more complicated, and therefore more highly reimbursed, will allow the surgeon to use these descriptions upfront. Knowing that there is a more appropriate code will allow for better compensation. You only need to know how to document to justify the code for which you are expecting to be paid.

Several decades ago, the most important part of billing was based on procedures done in the operating room. But reimbursement for operations has shrunk and patient management encounters have become more highly valued. Now, billing for each of the components of care has become more important. The relative value of a complex oncologic resection will always be higher than that of an office visit, but billing for all periods of care regardless of their relative worth can increase production by 20–40% and increase take-home pay by even more. Think of it as filling your basket with eggs. Some of those eggs may be worth a lot more than others, but if you spend your effort on only the high value eggs, you will miss the abundance of lower value ones. At the end of the day, you need to fill your basket and the value of each egg matters less than picking up every one available.

The following paragraphs will define and provide examples of various terms used in billing and coding. Sample surigcal scenarios with their appropriate CPT codes are used to illustrate the process. Do not get hung up on memorizing CPT codes, modifiers, etc. and focus instead on broader concepts.

RVUs, Billings and Collections

Any service performed can generate a bill to the patient or his or her insurance company. You send the bill with a description of the procedure (see CPT below), associated diagnosis (see ICD-10 below), and a charge. What you get paid though is almost never the entire charge. Historically charges were based on the highest amount that was likely to be paid and often have not changed or have increased within the last several years. However, the amount actually collected has gone down markedly. Billings measures the total amount billed while collections indicates the amount that is actually paid. When you sign a contract with an insurance company, you or your practice agrees to accept their fee schedule and generally be paid less than you are billing. Also, in some situations you may bill a patient but never be paid, particularly with uninsured patients. Billings are always higher than collections, and collections are based on payer mix. Payer mix refers to the relative percentage of privately insured, Medicare, Medicaid, and self-pay (uninsured) patients. Generally private insurances pay the most while self-pay patients pay the least. Medicare and Medicaid typically fall somewhere in between in terms of collections. Relative Value Units (RVUs) are nonmonetary measure of the value of a procedure or service. RVUs are useful as they do not vary with payer mix and represent a work value. They also allow comparison across specialties. Generally, the higher the RVU value the greater the reimbursement, but this is not a linear arrangement. Patient care services should not be disparaged as a billing source. If done correctly, these can earn as much as procedural billings. Average RVU production varies a great deal amongst different specialties, and specialties that generate higher RVU values are generally paid more. Specialties with higher salaries typically are paid a higher average dollar amount per RVU. Physicians are never paid solely by the number of hours worked.

CPT Codes

CPT is a five-digit code that represents a billable act of care. The complexity and difficulty of a procedure determines the appropriate CPT, which determines allowable charges and associated RVUs. CPT codes are not specialty specific, and the same procedure done by two different specialists is reimbursed the same amount. Most operative procedures have specific codes but for new or rare procedures an unlisted code can be used. Generally, it is better to pick the most appropriate code and use unlisted codes sparingly as unlisted codes reimburse inconsistently. Unlisted codes require a greater amount of documentation, do not reimburse as quickly and require a higher amount of administrative overhead to deal with denials or requests for more information. Moreover, most RVU-based reimbursement systems fail to recognize the work of procedures documented with unlisted codes as the unlisted code has no RVU valuation in the Centers for Medicare and Medicaid Services (CMS) database. However, for newer procedures, unlisted codes may be the only viable option to gain reimbursement.

There are codes for both Evaluation and Management (E&M) and procedures. Examples of E&M codes are those for office encounters, inpatient consults, and ED admissions. Further there are modifiers for these CPT codes that can do several things, including allowing you to bill multiple codes on the same day or within the global period. Some modifier codes allow for billing on the same day as the initial evaluation. CPT codes are grouped by procedure type with the following classes: 1xxxx for skin and soft tissue codes; 2xxxxx for orthopedics; 3xxxx for vascular codes; 4xxxx for gastrointestinal; 5xxxx for urology, gynecology, and endocrine; 6xxxxx for neurosurgery and ophthalmology; 7xxxx for radiologic interpretation; 8xxxxx for pathology and lab procedures; and 9xxxx for E&M. A general surgeon may use codes from all of the above categories, but skin, gastrointestinal, vascular, and E&M are the most frequently used. CPT codes must be linked to an ICD-10 code that represents the diagnosis for which the procedure or evaluation is performed.

Global Period

The care of patients after a procedure includes all appropriate postoperative treatments and is termed the global period. The length of the global period varies depending on the procedure performed. Endoscopy procedures have no global period. Minor procedures, such as removal of skin lesions, drainage of an abscess, mass removal, and other procedures that can generally be done in the office, have a 10 day global period. The location at which a procedure is performed does not change the global period. Resection of a skin cancer in the operating room has the same 10 day global period as a resection done in the office. Major procedures, generally those that are done in operating room, have a 90 day global period. The global period includes the 24 h prior to the procedure as well. For example, endoscopy procedures are considered zero day global codes, meaning that 24 h prior to the procedure and all events on the day of the procedure are included in the global period. Care unrelated to the primary problem is not included in the global period but documentation must make it clear that a seperate issue is being assessed and treated. Evaluation and Management (E&M) procedures done in the global period require an appropriate modifier. Also evaluation or treatment that is not part of the usual postoperative care is billable. This could include critical care delivered in the postoperative period or the treatment of complications not directly related to the procedure. This is where discussions with your coders become very helpful.

Modifiers

Modifiers are two-digit codes added to CPTs to clarify coding and often allow multiple codes to be billed on the same day of service or allow payments for CPTs billed within the global period. Common modifiers used in general surgery include the following:

Bilateral-50: Bilateral inguinal hernias are repaired. Bill 49505 and 49505-50. The first procedure is paid in full and the second at a reduced rate, usually 50%.

Decision for surgery-24 (office) or -57 (inpatient): This explains that you evaluated the patient and made a clinical decision to operate. Example: You see and evaluate a patient with right lower quadrant pain and decide to operate on them for appendicitis. The codes billed are 99222-57 and 47590. The E&M code otherwise is not paid on the day of surgery. You are not allowed to bill an E&M code on the day of an elective surgery when you update the history and physical.

Separate procedures-59: You perform two separate CPT codes on the same patient on the same day, generally this requires separate incisions. Example: You place a port-a-cath the same day as a laparoscopic right colectomy. As they are generally not done together or through same incision, you bill 44205 (lap right colectomy, primary procedure), and 36561-59 (port-a-cath insertion). The first procedure is paid in full and subsequent procedures are paid at a reduced rate that is state dependent. The better paying procedure should be billed without the modifier.

Return to OR staged (planned)-58: This covers procedures done within the global period after the initial operation when the subsequent operation is clearly planned. Example: You do an open breast biopsy that returns cancer, you return to OR in 7 days (within the global period) for a simple mastectomy. The appropriate codes are 19120 (open breast biopsy) on the day of the initial surgery and 19303-58 (simple mastectomy) on the day of the second surgery. This also covers if a subsequent procedure is significantly more involved than the initial surgery. Both procedures are paid in full.

Return to the OR for a related issue-78: This covers procedures in the global period not planned but requiring a return to the operation room clearly related to the primary procedure. Example: You evacuate a hematoma the day after an open inguinal hernia repair. 49505 (open inguinal hernia) is billed for the initial date of surgery and 10140-78 is billed for the return the next day. The second procedure is paid at a reduced rate, usually 50%.

Return to OR for unrelated issues-79: This covers procedures in the global period not planned but requiring a return to the operating room that is clearly not related to the primary procedure. Example: You electively repair a right inguinal hernia via a laparoscopic approach. The patient then returns 40 days later with peritonitis from a perforated ulcer. The original surgery is billed as 49650, lap inguinal hernia, and the subsequent surgery is billed as 44840-79 (Gastrorrhaphy, suture of perforation). Both are paid in full.

First assistant—FA: A qualified resident or fellow assistant is not available needs to be documented in note. A first assistant bills the same code as the primary surgeon with FA modifier to indicate he or she was serving as first assistant. This pays between 10–20% of primary procedure.

For a list of frequently used modifiers, see Appendix.

More Considerations for Major Operations

Major operations are billed on the most complex portion rather than each of the parts. An exploratory laparotomy for lysis of adhesions with bowel resection is billed only as a small bowel resection. Billing for each of these parts is considered unbundling. To maximize the efficiency of your billing, use the appropriate code for the most complex part of the operation. Avoid unspecified codes unless no other codes apply. Procedures occurring subsequently in the global period need appropriate modifiers and the choice of an appropriate modifier is reflected in the amount paid. A return to the operating room is paid at about 50% when it occurs in the global period unless the return is planned at the time of the original operation or is more extensive (in which case a modifier 58 is required). A laparoscopic procedure that is converted to open is billed as an open procedure.

Multiple procedures will pay 100% for the first code and less on each subsequent procedure. The percentage paid on each subsequent procedure varies from state to state. For procedures performed at the same visit by two or more different surgeons, each surgeon bills for his or her procedure independent of the other. For example, a right oophorectomy performed by a gynecologist at the same time as a lap appendectomy would each be paid in full. Procedures performed by the same surgeon via different incisions will often pay at half their value (for example, simultaneous right and left inguinal hernia repairs or a PEG at the same time as a port-a-cath placement). Add-on codes are special in that they pay in full in addition to the primary code, i.e., mobilization of the splenic flexure is an add-on code for left colon procedures. Placement of a feeding jejunostomy is another add-on code. Several of the procedures done by length or size have add-on codes to increase size. For example, in complex closure of 14 cm axillary wound, appropriate billing includes CPT 13132 (complex closure axillary wound 2.5–7.5 cm) and CPT 13133 billed twice (complex closure axillary wound additional length up to 5.0 cm).

For multiple endoscopic procedures, reimbursement is typically 50% for a procedure with a separate approach. Thus EGD would be paid at 50% if performed at the same time as a colonoscopy. Reimbursement for multiple endoscopic procedures with the same approach is more complex. For example, tattooing a lesion (CPT 45381) and snare polypectomy (CPT 45385) are paid as the stem procedure (diagnostic colonoscopy, CPT 45378) plus the difference between the stem and each of the other procedures (45385-45378 + 45381-45378). This amounts to a modest increase in what is reimbursed.

Hernia Billing

Hernia billing includes some special considerations regarding the differences between inguinal and ventral, laparoscopic and open, use of mesh in repair, patient's age, and status of hernia. First we will consider open hernia repairs. Open inguinal hernia CPTs always include mesh, if used, and are divided into reducible, incarcerated or non-reducible, and strangulated. They are further stratified by initial or recurrent with a separate category for sliding hernias. Finally inguinal hernia repairs in patients under 6 month of age, 6 months to 5 years old, and over 5 years old each have different CPT codes.

Open umbilical and epigastric hernia repairs have separate CPT codes that always include mesh and are separated only into reducible and nonreducible. Open incisional and ventral hernias are considered the same, but they are divided into initial or recurrent and reducible or nonreducible. Use of mesh is a separate add-on code (49568) for ventral and incisional hernia repair. Further, open repair using a retrorectus mesh and separation of components (TARS repair, for example) can be billed as the separation of components, (15734, myocutaneous flap, trunk) in addition to the hernia repair codes. Commonly both sides are mobilized so a bilateral muscle flap code is utilized. For example, a large reducible, incisional hernia repaired with bilateral transversus abdominis release and mesh placed in retrorectus space can be billed as 49560 (initial repair ventral or incisional hernia, reducible), 15734-59 (code and modifier for a myocutaneous flap) and 15734-50-59 (code and modifiers indicating a bilateral myocutaneous flap) and 49568 (add-on code for TAR). Finally, there is separate code for open repair of a Spigelian hernia.

Laparoscopic codes all include mesh, so an add-on code for mesh is not appropriate in these cases. Laparoscopic inguinal hernias are separated into initial and recurrent hernias. Laparoscopic umbilical, epigastric, Spigelian, and ventral hernias are all grouped together under two codes splitting reducible hernias from nonreducible. Laparoscopic repair of incisional hernias is divided into initial and recurrent repairs and again by reducibility.

Outpatient E&M Codes and Associated Minor Office-Based Procedures

There are separate codes for the initial evaluation and subsequent office visits for outpatients and for initial evaluation and subsequent daily charges for inpatients. Initial evaluations for clinic visits are subdivided into initial management codes (9920x) and consult codes (9924x). Consults pay better than equal level initial management codes but require specific documentation. The exact language used by both the requesting physician and the consulting physician is important. There has to be a request from another physician that uses the specific language of consultation or evaluation regarding a specific clinical problem or symptom. "Refer to Dr. Smith for gallstones" is not considered appropriate language of request to justify a consultation. The consult note must include the verbiage "Patient seen in consult at the request of Dr. Smith for x," and a copy of the consult note must be sent back to the physician requesting the consult. Neither Medicare nor Medicaid recognizes consult codes. Subsequent visits are billed using established patient codes (9921x). A patient who has not been seen in three years becomes a new patient from a billing standpoint.

Consult codes for a new problem can be applied to new or established patients. The codes are based on complexity and require documentation to justify each level. Documentation requirements break down into a minimum number of elements from HPI, ROS, exam, and past medical/family/social history elements. The elements of chief complaint include location, quality, severity, duration, timing, context, and modifying factors, and the number of elements required varies based on the level of billing (see Table 4.1).

For each of these different levels, there is a degree of complexity than should be documented. There is also a time requirement for each of these levels (Table 4.2). For surgeons, this is often the most straightforward means to document this

TABLE 4.1 New outpatient evaluations and outpatient consultations. Requirements for each element type based on level of billing

CPT code	HPI	ROS	Exam[a]	PMFSH
99201/99241	1	0	1	0
99202/99242	1	1	2	0
99203/99243	4	2	2	1
99204/99244	4	10	8	3
99205/99245	4	10	8	3

[a]For physical exam documentation, each arm counts as a separate area. Skin is also one area

TABLE 4.2 Office initial visit and consult: time requirement based on level and visit type

CPT code	Time requirement (in minutes)	
	Initial visit	Consult
99201/99241	10	15
99202/99242	20	30
99203/99243	30	40
99204/99244	45	60
99205/99245	60	80

level of complexity of care. Time spent in counseling/coordinating care, if at least 50% of the encounter length, can be used to justify the level complexity element. This means if you spend 30 min discussing how an operation is done and the risks/benefits, then you have justified the complexity for a level 4 consult or a level 5 new patient encounter. Consult codes always have a somewhat longer time requirement than initial visit codes, and often the next level of new patient encounter is nearly equivalent to the lower level consult code.

Office based procedures can be billed separately with a modifier 24 added to an E&M code. Common procedures include punch biopsy, removal of skin tumors (benign or malignant), mass removal, anoscopy, and abscess drainage. Two of these are more complex: the removal of skin lesions and subcutaneous mass removal.

Skin lesion excision is divided by benign and malignant lesions, the size of the lesion, and the area of the body. The size component is based on the width of the lesion including margins. The length of the incision does not matter. If the wound is closed in two layers, an intermediate wound closure code can be added which depends on the length of the wound and the area of the body.

For removal of masses below the skin, including lipomas and sebaceous cysts, billing is dependent on body area, mass size, and mass depth (subcutaneous versus below the fascia). These excisions are represented by 2xxxx codes, with there being four codes for each body area.

Inpatient E&M Codes and Procedures

Admission CPTs are divided into only 3 codes, 99231–99233, and, similar to outpatient visits, have associated HPI/ROS/ EXAM/PMFSH and time requirements that can be used to justify complexity. Level 1 admissions have fewer elements than level 2 or 3, which have the same required number of elements but differ in the time requirement (see Table 4.3).

Consult codes are broken into five levels with similar element and time requirements to the admission codes, as outlined in Table 4.4.

Subsequent visits are billed per day if the patient does not receive an operation. These can generate significant revenue particularly on trauma, critical care, and emergency general surgery services. Follow-up visits on consults and admissions are billed the same, and like the previously discussed codes, are based on complexity but also have required elements (see Table 4.5). Level 1 (99231) indicates an improving problem.

TABLE 4.3 Admission E&M: Element and time requirements for admission CPTs based on billing level

CPT code	HPI	ROS	EXAM	PMFSH	Time
99231	4	2	2	1	30 min
99232	4	10	8	3	50 min
99233	4	10	8	3	70 min

TABLE 4.4 Hospital inpatient consultation: Element and time requirements for inpatient consults based on billing level

CPT code	HPI	ROS	EXAM	PMFSH	Time
99251	1	0	1	0	20 min
99252	1	2	1	0	40 min
99253	4	2	2	1	55 min
99254	4	10	8	3	80 min
99255	4	10	8	3	110 min

TABLE 4.5 Inpatient follow-up

CPT code	HPI	Exam	ROS	Time
99231	1	1	0	15 min
99232	1	2	1	25 min
99233	4	2	2	35 min

Level 2 (99232) is used for a stable but not resolving issue, and level 3 (99233) demonstrates significant deterioration of the patient's condition. Hospital discharges can also be billed. Code 99238 is appropriate for discharges taking less than 30 min while 99239 are used for discharges taking longer than 30 min.

Differences with Medicare and Medicaid

There is generally little difference for Medicare and Medicaid in terms of coding except for a few instances for surgeons. Medicare and Medicaid no longer recognize consultation codes and all inpatient and outpatient encounters are billed using new patient or established patient codes on the outpatient side, and patient admission and follow-up codes on the inpatient side. Medicare and Medicaid use a special code for screening colonoscopies, G0121 for normal risk patients, and G0105 for high-risk patients instead of more typical 45378 used by private insurance companies. This last item is not often fixed by coders and is not something most surgeons need to know. Medicare is different from other insurances in that it offers the option of being a participating provider and agreeing to their fee schedule that is 5% higher than that for a nonparticipating provider. Nonparticipating providers can charge a higher overall fee however. Medicare as the insuring agent pays less to a nonparticipating provider and the higher overall fee is generated by billing the balance to the patient. Medicare still limits the overall charge to 115% of their fee schedule. The choice to not participate exists only in the private practice model, though in theory larger organizations could decide not to participate.

ICD-10

Diagnoses are specified by ICD-10 codes. ICD codes stand for International Statistical Classification of Diseases and Related Health Problems. ICD-10 refers to the newest iteration (10th Edition) that went into effect in the United States in October of 2015. It had been around for 10 years prior to its adoption. It effectively changed the base 13,000 codes in ICD-9 to 68,000 codes in ICD-10. ICD-9 was over 25 years old and medicine has changed significantly. ICD-10 allows for more specificity in coding. For those not familiar with ICD-9, this probably has not been much of an issue. However, this new coding system completely changed all codes, so those who were familiar with common codes are now left searching for their new counterparts. ICD-10 requires information about laterality, if an encounter is initial or subsequent, and more details of the condition. Electronic medical records make this transition much easier.

Starting Practice

Starting to practice in a new location requires several steps to allow you to be paid. The initial step is obtaining licensure from the state medical board and the DEA. You also need to obtain an NPI number (National Provider Identifier) which is a unique ten-digit number and is used by both Medicare/Medicaid as well as private insurance. Both state and DEA licenses can take several months to obtain, and certain states, Florida and Texas for example, take even longer and have significantly stricter licensure requirements. Only after you have both of these licenses can you apply for privileges at the hospitals at which you will be admitting, seeing consults and operating. This also can take several months to process as they go back to at least medical school and obtain records. Every place you work subsequently increases the length of the process. Also, as a provider you will need to sign contracts with each of the insurance companies prior to seeing any patient covered by them. So the entire process from signing a new contract to actually being able to see patients and bill for your services is at least 3 months and often 6 months. Sometimes services can be billed retroactively or under your partner's name.

Test your Knowledge

1. An elderly patient is seen in the emergency room with free air in the abdomen, sepsis, and multiple medical comorbidities. You evaluate the patient, review the labs and CT images, and discuss operative plans and options with patient and his family. You document in your admission H&P 4 elements of history, 10 ROS, 8 exam, and 3 PMFSH and that you spent 35 min discussing with the patient and his family and coordinating care. You go to operating room and perform exploratory laparotomy, resection of the sigmoid colon, and creation of an end colostomy. You mobilize the splenic flexure to allow the colostomy to reach an ideal site and place a feeding jejunostomy. What are the appropriate codes/level of billing?

2. True or False: A plastic surgeon who does a local flap procedure will get paid more than a general surgeon doing same procedure?

3. True or False: I remove the gallbladder of a patient, and a gynecologist comes in at end of the procedure and removes an ovary. I should bill just for the cholecystectomy and will get paid the same amount as it were done as an isolated procedure.

4. True or False: I can bill for an H&P on the day of surgery for a patient I originally saw in the office and scheduled for an elective procedure.

5. True or False: I can bill for an admission from the ER and an operation on the same day for a patient seen for the first time that day.

6. You see a patient in the office with a prior punch biopsy showing squamous cell cancer on two areas: the left upper arm and

the right thigh. You evaluate the patient, perform a basic history and exam, and recommend removal of both skin cancers at that same visit. The left arm lesion is 3 cm long and 1.7 cm wide on the upper arm. The right thigh lesion is 5 mm and round. You remove the left arm lesion with an elliptical incision 8 cm long by 2.8 cm wide and repair this in two layers, and excise the right thigh lesion via a 4 cm by 1.3 cm ellipse which is also repaired in two layers. What do you bill?

Test your Knowledge

1. 99223-57 (level 3 admission with a decision to operate modifier), 44143 Colectomy with end colostomy (primary procedure), 44139 Mobilize Splenic Flexure (add-on code), 44015 Tube or Needle Jejunostomy (second add-on code)
2. False, CPT is independent of specialty.
3. True, and note no modifier is required. There is a two surgeons modifier if two surgeons are required to complete a procedure, but as each surgeon in this example has a separate CPT and separate diagnosis, each is billed as they are independent events.
4. False, the decision to operate was made already in the office. Even if you produce a new History and Physical, this is part of operation billing that day.
5. True. Like number one, you needed to evaluate and decide if an operation was appropriate.
6. 99201-24 (level 1 new patient with decision to operate), 11063 (excise malignant skin lesion of trunk, arm, or leg, 2.1–3.0 cm), 11062-57 (excise malignant skin lesion of trunk, arm, or leg, 1.1–2.0 cm with separate procedure modifier), 12034-57 (intermediate repair of incision 7.6–12.5 cm of arm, leg, scalp, or trunk). Note each lesion removed is listed separately even though they are in the same "body area," but an intermediate repair is the sum of all repairs for a given body area, with body area defined by ICD-10. If you had removed a lesion from the patient's face instead of the right thigh, then a separate code for intermediate repair of the face would be appropriate.

Final Tips

Billing between the anesthesia and the surgeon need to match, otherwise the second bill to arrive will not initially be paid. Some surgeons tell the anesthesiologist the codes at end of procedure, which often they appreciate.

Working with your coder is an invaluable learning experience and can increase understanding for both the surgeon and the coder. The coder is one of the most important of your employees. They require ongoing education as rules for coding change constantly.

The last example showed 4–5 codes that could be used for two skin cancers. It is less important that you know that each can be billed for independently and the exact CPTs used. It is more important that you document the width, including margins, of each lesion, whether it is benign or malignant, and the location from which it was excised. A coder can then fill in the details. In similar fashion, it is less important to know the skin closure codes than to know what constitutes a simple, intermediate, or complex closure and the need to document the total length.

There is no way you will remember all of these CPT codes. Having a CPT manual written by the AMA in the operating room and office is very helpful. A good substitute is a coding app for your smartphone called **ABEO coder** that is available for free. This app was designed for anesthesiologists but is very useful tool. Descriptions are more limited than those in the AMA manual but still very useful, and it allows you to save your favorite codes.

Further references include basic and advanced coding workshops, website and hotline, all sponsored by the American College of Surgeons.

Coding courses: https://www.facs.org/advocacy/practmanagement/workshops

Coding bulletins and hotline: https://www.facs.org/advocacy/practmanagement/cpt

Appendix

Frequently used modifiers for surgical billing

Code	Use	Example
-24	For evaluation and management of a problem unrelated to the primary diagnosis completed within the global period	A patient who has previously undergone a hernia repair returns within the global period with complaint of biliary colic
-25	For evaluation and management of a problem unrelated to the reason for a procedure completed on the same day as the procedure	A patient presents for removal of a skin lesion with a new onset right groin pain
-50	To indicate bilaterality	A right inguinal hernia repair completed on the same day as a left hernia repair (only one CPT will carry this modifier)
-53	To indicate the procedure was aborted prior to completion	A patient develops an allergic reaction to local anesthetic requiring the planned hernia repair be aborted. An operative note must be submitted indicating why the procedure was aborted and at what step.
-57	For evaluation and management of the primary problem if originally diagnosed on the same day as a procedure	The workup of a patient in the Emergency Department who later goes to the OR for an appendectomy

-58	For a planned take back or staged procedure when this procedure is completed within the global period	A mastectomy that takes place within the global period of previously completed open breast biopsy
-59	To indicate a separate and unrelated procedure that was completed on the same day as the primary procedure	A port-a-cath placement completed at the same time as PEG placement
-78	To indicate an unplanned return to the OR related to the primary procedure	A patient develops fascial dehiscence after a laparotomy requiring return to the OR for exploration and fascial closure
-79	For an unplanned return to the OR unrelated to the original procedure	A patient who underwent inguinal hernia repair develops appendicitis within the global period

Chapter 5
Military and Government Practice

COL. Robert B. Lim and Stanley Zagorski

Introduction

Considering a career in government service as a physician is another possible career path one that can be rewarding and satisfying for different reasons including fulfilling a sense of patriotism. The options are joining the military on Active Duty service or becoming a Government Service (GS) employee and working in a Veterans Administration (VA) hospital or a military treatment facility (MTF) as a civilian. There are many advantages and disadvantages between both options when compared to a civilian practice. This chapter will discuss the aspects of joining and leaving government service. The purpose of this chapter is to help guide the surgeon into government service and into the civilian sector once their government service is over.

C.R.B. Lim, M.D., F.A.C.S., F.A.S.M.B.S. (✉)
Department of Surgery, Tripler Army Medical Center,
1 Jarrett White Road, Honolulu, HI 96859, USA
e-mail: Robert.b.lim.mil@mail.mil

S. Zagorski, M.D., F.A.C.S.
Conemaugh Memorial Medical Center, Johnstown, PA

© Springer International Publishing AG 2017   69
D.B. Renton et al. (eds.), *The SAGES Manual Transitioning to Practice*, DOI 10.1007/978-3-319-51397-3_5

Working on Active Duty

Most physicians who work on Active Duty do so because they used a military scholarship to pay for medical school, the Health Professionals Scholarship Program (HPSP), or by attending the military's medical school at the Uniformed Services University of the Health Sciences (USUHS). Some may have incurred time due to a scholarship to pay for undergraduate school, the Reserved Officer Training Corps (ROTC) scholarship, or they attended one of the service academies like the United States Military Academy at West Point. For those who have chosen this path, there are few military requirements during medical school. One is to attend the Officer Basic Course for Medical Corps officers, which typically occurs between the 1st and 2nd years of medical school. It is a 6-week course and one is considered on temporary Active Duty for the course, consequently travel, lodging, and a salary are paid for by the Department of Defense (DOD). So it's like having a summer job. The second requirement is that two of the fourth year electives have to be done at a MTF, which most medical students use as an extended interview. They typically choose electives based on where they would like to attend residency.

Those persons who have a military obligation through HPSP, ROTC, USUHS, or from attending a service academy are required to apply for residency in a military residency program. There is a match process for this process, which is similar to the civilian match system [1]. Payback for the scholarship would not start until once residency is finished; but during residency, they would be considered on Active Duty and this time does count towards retirement. So if one did a 6-year residency, they would need 14 more years on Active Duty to be eligible for the retirement benefits. During this time, in addition to earning basic pay that is based on one's rank, they will also earn a Basic Allowance for Housing (BAH) and Basic Allowance for Sustenance (BAS). Some may also earn a Cost of Living Allowance (COLA) based on where the residency is located. Except for basic pay, all of these are tax-free and they can increase with rank and the number of dependents (spouse and children). Additionally, they will be eligible for medical and dental care. All of this means, military residents will earn more money than their civilian counterparts.

US citizens also have the option to join Active Duty once their residency is complete and they are eligible for board certification. Here, there is no obligation incurred other than the initial contract one signs to join the military. Those who choose this option will have to attend Officer Basic Course immediately after they enter Active Duty so they can become accustomed to military regulations, like how to wear the uniform properly, and protocol, like how and when to salute. There are a few bonuses that one is eligible for after joining. The Active Duty Health Professions Loan Repayment Program gives the recipient $120 K and the Health Professions Special Pay gives $75 K. A bonus will typically require one to owe more years of service. Their residency does not count towards retirement.

Regardless of how one enters into the military, after residency and the Officer Basic Course have been completed, military physicians will be assigned to a duty station. This placement is based on the needs of the military. While one can submit a wish list, there is no guarantee they will be assigned their desired location. The decision is based on the needs of the military and can be greatly influenced by someone who is not even a physician. So if one wanted to only do advanced laparoscopic foregut cases after finishing residency, for instance, they may be assigned to a remote base where there is not much need for that kind of service or the MTF is not equipped for that type of surgery. This may also affect one's spouse too, as they may have to change the location of their job. The physician should be aware again that he or she may not have much choice regarding this.

After residency has been completed, one will have achieved the rank of an O-3 or O-4, which currently has a basic pay salary of about $47,000–53,400. This will increase every 2 years while on Active Duty. The DOD always pays for relo-

TABLE 5.1 Starting salary for O-3–O-4[a]

Type of pay	O-3–O-4 amount annually ($)
Basic pay	47,000–53,400
Basic allowance for housing	12,300–17,700
Basic allowance for sustenance	3000
Variable specialty pay	5000–12,000
Medical additional special pay	15,000
Board certification pay	2400–6000
Incentive specialty pay	20,000–36,000
Total	**$104,700–143,100.00**

[a]O-3 is a Captain in the Army and Air Force and a Lieutenant in the Navy. O-4 is a Major in the Army and Air Force and a Lieutenant Commander in the Navy

cation while on Active Duty whether one graduated from West Point and attended USUHS or one just joined the military. The cost of taking board examinations will also be covered. Additionally they will be eligible for more pay and bonuses. Physicians will annually receive Medical Additional Special Pay (MASP), which is a yearly lump sum of $15 K and Variable Special Pay (VSP), which is about $5–12 K annually. Once they become board certified, they will qualify for Board Certified Pay (BCP), about $2.4–6 K annually, and Incentive Specialty Pay (ISP), which is up to $36 K annually depending on the specialty. They will still earn the aforementioned tax-free BAH, BAS, and COLA. All told, the military surgeon will make a salary ranging about $105,000–143,000. This is likely to be quite a bit less than those in the civilian environment where the average starting salary is $226,000 [2] (see Table 5.1).

The latter salary does not, however, take into account taxes, overhead costs, medical school loan payback, and liability insurance. The taxable income for military physicians will be less than that of civilian ones and government physicians do not pay liability insurance. When claims of medical malpractice are made, the claim goes against the US government and any payout is made by the US government. The physician is only listed as a witness and the court rules on whether or not the US government is liable. The physician can still be found to have not met the standard of care in malpractice cases, but this is not determined by the court. As such, the physician can still be placed in the National Practitioner's Databank.

There is no overhead cost for government doctors to practice. As mentioned before, medical and dental benefits are free for the service member and his or her dependents. Also, as a military service member, one is eligible for a VA home loan meaning a new home can be purchased, up to a certain limit depending on the area of the country, without a down payment, though there is about a 1% VA funding fee. This tends to make these salaries closer but it is also specialty and location dependent. For the pediatricians and primary care providers, the guaranteed money in the military may be substantially more than that in the civilian sector. Conversely, a surgeon in a smaller, low cost-of-living community will likely make a lot more money than the military surgeon.

Another advantage of all government service is that pay is not dependent on productivity. So the lifestyle may not be as demanding as it is in the private sector. There are federal holidays to honor and all military employees get 30 days of paid leave every year.

The disadvantages, though, are prevalent. The biggest one is deployments. Unfortunately these are unpredictable and since general surgeons are the experts in trauma surgery, they are the most deployed of all the medical specialties. It is an honor to serve on deployments; but there is no doubt that it is a significant interruption in one's surgical practice. A recent graduate can expect to deploy within 1 year of finishing his or her residency and then every 2 years thereafter for as long as there is conflict in which the United States has troops deployed. Aside from being apart from their family, there is a risk of dying in combat albeit relatively small. Three surgeons have died in combat since the wars in Afghanistan and Iraq started in 2001. Even in the quietest of deployments to the combat zone, most surgeons have experienced indirect if not direct fire. Additionally, one may still feel the strain of the deployment even if one has not been selected to go. The providers left behind will have to cover the work of the one who has deployed, which often means more call and more administrative tasking.

After the deployment has been served, reintegration back into regular practice can be problematic. The first few complex laparoscopic cases or complex breast cancer case may cause a lot of anxiety after spending 6 months in the desert doing only a few trauma cases. It is best to have a more senior surgeon assist with those cases and those decision-making processes. If one is not available in the MTF, often times, the local civilian hospital may have an agreement in place to assist with this. Surgical societies like the American College of Surgeons (ACS) and the Society of American Gastrointestinal and Endoscopic Surgeons (SAGES) have recognized this issue, and have begun implementing programs to have a mentor, within the nearby civilian community, available to the MTFs. In rare cases, the new residency graduate may have to draft a memorandum that outlines the working and legal relationship between the two hospitals that allows such a relationship.

While on Active Duty, those who would like to pursue an academic career have to do so on their free time. There are fewer resources to complete studies and no administrative help. Additionally there is no extra incentive to publish. Being a Professor of Surgery in the military does not afford one any more pay or status within the military.

Another issue will be the administrative load. At least some of the workweek will be dedicated to completing the many administrative tasks of the military. Having a leadership position has its advantages and disadvantages. While it is nice to have the title for one's resume, often times these positions will be assumed with one having very little management experience or operational knowledge. There are a lot of personnel, supply, and management decisions that need attention in order to run a clinic. This, of course, adds to the administrative work, detracts from one's clinical time, and does not incur a pay raise. At a time when the young surgeon is supposed to grow from being competent to proficient, a leadership position may halt or delay that progression. It is imperative, therefore, for the young surgeon to recognize when his or her clinical skills are waning. Those who plan to stay 20 years and desire promotion will need to take the Captain's Career Course and the Intermediate Level Education Course, both of which will take a physician away from their practice for several months. It should also be noted that if one has aspirations of becoming a Flag Officer (a General or an Admiral) then they will have to abandon clinical practice altogether after about 10–12 years of service to assume administrative and operational commands. It is distinct success in the leadership and command positions that will get one promoted to the highest level. Academic achievement and publication success will have little to no influence on promotion.

Finally, the clinician will not be her own boss. In addition to events like the semiannual physical fitness tests, there will be a lot of mandatory military training like how to react in case of a chemical and biological weapons attack or cyber security classes. Failure to complete these tasks may result in a negative credentialing action against the provider. Also, funding for Continuing Medical Education (CME) is very limited for military physicians and many end up of paying for keeping up their education out of their own pocket. This can be very frustrating for one who has deployed for 6 months and then attended a military course for another 4 months.

If one plans to serve for more than 3 years in the military, likely they will be reassigned to another duty station. While there is a consultant, who is a physician in their specialty, for each medical specialty to help decide duty assignments, the Human Resources Command (HRC) will have a lot of influence on where the next assignment occurs. Again the HRC will have the military's best interest in mind not the physician's, and thus, someone who is not even a physician or a clinician may make the surgeon's life-altering decision. It will not be uncommon to encounter a physician who was moved abruptly and against their desires, often times at hardship to their family or to the detriment of the practice they have built, and despite a senior rank, a sterling academic resume, and a unique surgical skill set. It goes without saying that such a decision can be very disheartening for the military physician.

Most persons who incur a military obligation through the scholarship programs will be accustomed to these aspects of military life so hopefully; this won't be a surprise to these surgeons. Still it is a lot to consider when making a decision after residency is complete and a very difficult one to make when one is deciding on how to pay for medical school. The work can be very rewarding as providing trauma care on soldiers who have been injured in battle is much different than operating on someone who was drunk and got into a bar fight. Additionally after 20 years of service, the retirement plan would pay an annuity that increases with inflation for each year of their life after they leave military service on top of whatever job they took until finally deciding to stop working altogether. The finances of the pension will be discussed later in more detail.

Working as a Government Service Employee or Veterans Administration Employee

As a GS employee, a physician would be taking care of active duty service members, dependents, and retirees in an MTF. Those who opt for the VA healthcare system would be caring for retirees and those service members whose medical illness was due to their military duty. The main advantages to joining are similar to that of joining the military: steady income not entirely based on production, less pressure to produce, no overhead including liability insurance, a better lifestyle, and for some, the opportunity to fulfill their patriotic sense of duty. Not everyone can serve on Active Duty and deploy to care for military members, joining as a government worker allows them to still serve their country.

The VA and GS employee salaries are based on a given grade level and each grade has ten steps. The grade is based on the scope, complexity, and work performed on a range from 1 to 15 with the higher numbers being more complex. Within the grade, there are ten steps with each step corresponding to an increase in salary of about 3%. A board of physicians within the VA determines this and most physicians will eventually qualify for the tenth step. Upon entering the VA system, though, a physician is started at a GS-15 grade, step 1. Some physicians that are highly specialized or who have previous time in the government will start at a higher step. In addition to this base salary, there is a locality pay which is additional pay based on percentage of the salary decided by location. The percentage in 2016 will range from about 14–35 %. A general surgeon who is a GS-15, step 10 will make a base salary of about $132,000. With the addition of locality pay of an additional $18,500–46,200, this would be about $150,000–178,000 [3]. The VA does have a 1-year probationary period, so that if things are not working out, the employee can be released or opt out of service.

Further salary is then based on market pay and performance pay. The market pay is simply what the need of the VA system is based on recruitment and retention of physicians in the same field. Market pay is highly variable and can be substantial to make the salary more attractive to surgeons. Performance pay is intended to reward the achievement of goals and objectives that are set forth by an annual appraisal. Like the military, there will be a regular pay raise as more years of service are completed. In the end, the salary for a VA general surgeon can range from about $150,000–$355,000 based on years of service, location, and market value [4].

The GS employee enjoys the similar military benefits in that liability insurance and overhead costs are not needed. Unlike Active Duty surgeons, medical and dental benefits are not free but coverage is provided. GS employees have the option of not taking this coverage. Every 2 weeks of work earns one day of leave, so he or she is eligible for 26 days of leave per year. There are also loan repayment and retention programs that would obligate the surgeon to more years of service. One advantage GS employment has over Active Duty service is that one can choose where they would like to work and there is no requirement to move every 3 years.

The disadvantage of GS employment is also similar to that of the military. While one won't be required to move every 2–3 years or be deployed, one will not likely be their own boss. There will be administrative tasks, nonclinical requirements, and non-clinicians dictating the practice. Ultimately, the individual would have to decide how important this is to him or her. Another issue with the VA system and to a certain extent in the military system is availability of services to the beneficiaries. Not every town has a VA hospital and thus eligible patients may have to travel long distances for fairly routine services like a laparoscopic cholecystectomy. This can be frustrating to both the patient and the providers. Additionally if certain services are not available at the VA, like a gastroenterologist who does endoscopic ultrasound, this may have to be referred to another provider, which may significantly delay the process until definitive care can be done [5]. Finally and anecdotally, there exists the stigma that there are physicians in the government systems that are just there to collect a paycheck until they are eligible for a pension. Since their work is not based on efficiency or productivity and they have seniority or perhaps, even a leadership position, he or she may not be the best clinician to have as a partner. There is no documentation of this, of course, and there is no reason to believe that it is widespread. When provider tenure is not based on productivity, this can be a natural sequel. It should be noted, however, that there are several studies that report good quality outcomes in the VA system [6].

Overall, whether one joins the military or becomes a GS employee, the quality of life may be more comfortable with reliable pay. The type of patients one serves may be more rewarding but the overall job satisfaction may be lower. Military life also has the added issues of deployment, frequent moves, frequent changes in leadership and leadership policies, and increased administrative requirements. In the end, though, there will still be of opportunities to practice surgery and develop into a good clinician.

Leaving Government Service

Leaving government service to start work in the civilian world is quite different than graduating from residency or changing jobs early in one's career. For one thing, most of these surgeons have been practicing for several years, are board certified, and even held a position of leadership. They are typically at a different stage in life, perhaps with a mortgage or with children who are ready to start high school or college. At the same time, GS employees have not typically had to follow the same metrics and standards that civilian surgeons have had to regarding reimbursement, productivity, and overhead cost. Moreover, they have not had to be concern with the cost of liability insurance. As such, they may have different expectations for their job and pay in the civilian world. In some aspects, they could be an expert but in others, they can be as unaware as the graduating Chief Resident.

Even if one is not leaving for financial reasons, there are financial aspects that one must consider. One, the tax-free BAH, BAS, and COLA are no longer available. Henceforth, all of their earned money will be taxed. This increase in one's taxable total income will likely put them in a higher tax bracket. On the other hand, if one had bought a house using the VA loan and then sells the home when they leave government service, they are eligible to use the same VA loan again, and thus they can purchase a new home with no down payment again. These aspects must be considered to help one decide on what kind of civilian job to take and how much salary they need to continue with their current standard of living.

When to Get Out of the Military

For those in military service, this is likely a very big question. The decision to leave the military has many opinions and is based on many factors; but most will agree that it should not be based on money alone. Most financial planners will also agree that leaving the military after ten or more years of ser-

TABLE 5.2 Monthly retirement pay per rank[a,b]

	O-3 ($)	O-4 ($)	O-5 ($)	O-6 ($)	O-7 ($)
20 years	3224.04	3763.32	4308.44	4923.86	6161.33
22 years	3546.44	4139.65	4882.00	5558.78	6777.43
24 years	3707.65	4515.98	5325.82	6221.52	7393.60
26 years	4191.25	4892.32	5769.63	7070.53	8050.51
28 years	4513.66	5268.65	6213.45	7614.42	8669.78
30 years	4836.06	5644.98	6657.27	8321.23	9474.91

[a]This is 50% of the base pay. Rates are subject to change and are based on 2016 projections
[b]The retirement pay is actually based on the average monthly salary of the last 3 years of service. These rates will vary as may the time in rank amongst individuals

vice is not financially savvy for the majority of physicians. For one, there is no retirement plan that can match the current one offered for military service. After 20 years of service, the military offers an annual annuity at 50% of the average of the service member's last 3 years of pay. As mentioned before, this annuity also increases with inflation. Most physicians will retire as an O-5 or O-6, which means their retirement pay will be about $51,700–59,100 annually (See Table 5.2). Additionally, the retirement package also includes lifelong medical and dental coverage. If one estimates this to cost about $2000.00 monthly or about $24,000.00 annually, this means the annuity for this retirement package pays about $75,000–83,000 annually. This alone is not enough to live the way one may be accustomed to living but this certainly brings added financial security as collection for this retirement pay starts as soon as one retires from the military and not at age 62 or 65. An O-5 officer who serves 20 years would earn $4308.44 monthly which would cover the mortgage of a $700,000 home, using the VA loan with no down payment and a 4.0% interest rate over 30 years.

So one financial question for those deciding to get out before retirement is how much money does one have to invest in a pension to match the cost of losing out on the military's retirement plan? This has a lot of variables but assume that the surgeon wants to leave after her 10th year of service. At that point she will likely be an O-4 making approximately $160,000 annually of which about $20,000.00 is tax-free. If she would like to have that same $74,000 annually, one assumes a market rate of return on their pension investment of about 6%, and one uses only 3–5% of their money to have for retirement at 65, then the estimated amount of investment needed is anywhere from $6200–11,000 per month or $74,400–132,000 for 10 years. This assumes a 1% inflation rate and no change in investment plans if the market return goes below 6%. This means one would need to earn an extra $74,000–132,000 annually that would all go towards their retirement pension plan. So she would need a position that pays $234,000–292,000 annually if all of that additional pay went to retirement investment. This also assumes she would like to start collecting this pay 10 years after she leaves the military, which most physicians would not typically do.

According to one website, the salary of a general surgeon ranges from $249,700-336,000 [7], which one might think will be more than enough to pay for a retirement plan similar to the military's. Remember, though, that this new salary will be taxed at 33% (married filed jointly) v a 25% rate since the amount of taxable income is less [8]. This makes the net civilian salary about $167,299–225,120. There will also be more overhead cost, like liability insurance that for the average general surgeon is about $15,000 annually, so now the net salary is closer to $152,299–210,120. While the salary after taxes for the military surgeon is around $140,000, one can see there is not as much difference as initially thought especially if one would like a similar pension plan. The pay difference is not as significant and while the higher end of the civilian general surgeon's salary is significant, those types of jobs are not available in every location where one might want to live. Ultimately to make up the difference of those 10 years, one would have to get a job that after taxes pays that $234,000–292,000 with all of that extra money going toward the retirement investment. Since most physicians are not retiring at age 46, what this really means is that they will have to work longer and invest a lot more to match the pension plan of the military.

Conversely if one were to stick it out in the military for 20 years and then assume a surgeon's job, they would also have the additional $75,000–83,000 in annual income. Additionally the military does have the Multi-year Specialty Pay (MSP), which is a retention bonus that is available for those who have completed their initial military obligation. For general surgeons, this ranges from a 2-year contract at $60,000 per year to a 4-year contract at $110,000 per year. Combined with the pay raises that occur with more years of service and an increase in rank, the annual military salary will not be $100,000 less than the average general surgeon salary anymore. Again, financially, it may be best to stay in the military if one has already invested 10 years. It should be noted, though, that pay scales, pay raises, and retention bonuses are determined by Congress and are thus subject to change occassionally.

Like the military, GS employees enjoy a pension-related incentive package for years of service. Here it is called the FERS or Federal Employees Retirement System. It is a three tiered plan based on Social Security Benefits, FERS basic benefits, and the Thrift Savings Plan (TSP), which is similar to a 401 K. Unlike Active Duty surgeons, these monies are deducted from the GS employee's salary. Just like a 401 K, the employee can decide how much they want to allot to their TSP but the FERS and Social Security benefits are automatically deducted from their pay. The pension, like the military's, will be similar but here, 25 years of service affords one a pension plan with annuities based on the average of the highest three annual salaries of the provider while in government service. Another main difference is that the annuity is based on 25% of their total annual salary and not 50% of the base salary as it is in the military [9]. For the person who works long enough to earn a $355,000 annual salary, this would mean a monthly annuity of about $7400.

This, of course, is only considering the benefit of the government's pension programs. While the market dictates the salary, it is probably safe to say that most civilian pediatricians and primary care providers cannot compete with the pension plan provided by retiring from the military and or government service. Conversely, some bariatric surgeons and orthopedic surgeons probably can make more than enough to offset the tax breaks, the health insurance package, and the pension of retirement. For most others, though, the decision to stay in will come down to whether or not they care to deploy, and they care about career development, family stability, practice freedom, and the hassles of working for the government. If one has only 4–8 years invested in the military, then it may not be worth 12 years of deployments, moves, and following someone else's directives to stay for those remaining years.

Another aspect to consider is what kind of clinical surgery practice one wants after leaving the military. After 15–20 years in the military (including residency), one would be 40–45 years old. This is considered a senior surgeon in the military, and thus, one would likely have a position of leadership. This is quite often independent of clinical ability and if one spends the last 3–4 years of their military career doing mostly administrative work, they might be limiting their ability to perform robust clinical work. It would be quite rare for someone on Active Duty to be doing 400 or more cases per year even in the busiest of MTFs, unless they were also doing locum tenems work also. So if one would like to be a busy, technically superior surgeon and not an academic or administrative one, it would behoove them to try and avoid some leadership positions or administrative tasking that are commonplace for higher-ranking officers. If one cannot avoid this or prefers to eliminate the chance of this happening altogether, it may be wise to leave the military despite the retirement benefits.

Leaving the Military

Whether you leave after 6 years or leave after 20, most people in the military will recommend that one start planning for life after the military 2 years before the date of their retirement or release from the military. Like many young surgeons, recently graduated residents, or fellows, one of the first things the surgeon must do is decide on what type of job he or she wants. The general options are clinical only, academic and clinical, and resident based or resident affiliated. The surgeon should also decide on what type of surgeries they would like to mostly perform. For a general surgeon, for instance, would they like to do all of general surgery or would they like to specialize more, use robot-assisted laparoscopic surgery, do endoscopy, do trauma, or breast disease. Next, they should decide what type of practice they would like to be in: private practice, employed by the hospital, large group, or small group. This will have bearing on call frequency, call responsibilities, and clinic responsibilities. One should also decide what region of the country they would like to be in, the size of the city they where they would like to work, and an expectation for compensation.

Joining the VA after Active Duty is also an option and will add to their time of government service. As many VA hospitals are in need of leadership positions and are affiliated with an academic institution, this could be a viable option for those interested in administrative work or academics. It should be noted that if one leaves the military but continues on in government service in the VA or as a GS provider, they cannot collect their retirement pay and a separate salary from the government at the same time. Their years in the VA or as a GS employee though will contribute to their overall pension once they decide to leave government service completely.

If one later decides to return on Active Duty or return to the VA system, their previous service time is added on towards retirement. In other words, if someone serves 10 years in the military, enters a civilian practice, then returns to Active Duty 5 years later, he or she would already have 10 years towards retirement and would only have to serve ten more to make it to 20. Conversely some may opt to serve in the Reserves after finishing Active Duty. This too can be added to their current time in government and afford one more pay after they retire from service completely [10].

Those who elect to leave the military should utilize the Transition Assistance Program (TAP) to help them with the transition out of military life. All persons who served on Active Duty will have a percentage of disability evaluation by the VA medical system. In other words, if one develops chronic back pain due to a deployment-related injury, then he or she would be eligible to have the care for this injury covered by the VA system. This may affect benefits to them even if they have not served 20 years in the military, as the amount of disability directly affects pay earned. Here one must determine their level of physical health and what, if any, ailments will be eligible for treatment through the VA. During the process they will have a retirement physical and a Board will meet to determine how much of their ailments are eligible for this benefit. If this disability is combat-related or if the retiree has a 50% or greater disability, then this disability benefit is tax-free. For those that do retire from the military, the disability benefit since 2004 is given in addition to retirement pay [11]. One other retirement benefit is that for those retirees who have more than 10% disability, the VA funding fee for the VA home loan is waived.

There are many other financial things to remember prior to leaving Active Duty. Allotments to investments or to other financial institutions will automatically stop when one leaves the military. Retirees can arrange for their allotments to be taken from their retirement pay. But not all allotments will be transferrable from retirement pay; so one should discuss this with their Finance Office before leaving government service. Those that were on Active Duty after the events that occurred on September 11, 2001 are also eligible for the Post 9-11 GI Bill, which pays up to 36 months of educational benefits payable up to 15 years after the release from Active Duty. This benefit may be passed along to one's spouse, one's child or spread amongst their children to help pay for college as most physicians are not in need of this type of education. Naming these beneficiaries must occur before one leaves

Active Duty [12]. Government physicians do not need to have tail coverage insurance for the patients they cared for while in government service, because again any claim would go against the US government and not the individual provider.

Another aspect to consider for those that retire from the military is impending death. Life insurance can be complicated. All Active Duty members have Servicemembers Group Life Insurance (SGLI) that pays a lump sum of $500,000 to the beneficiaries in the event of death while on Active Duty. This benefit stops once Active Duty service has ended. Service members have the option of changing to Veterans Group Life Insurance (VGLI), which pays a maximum of $400,000 in coverage. The insurance question is a very detailed one, but if a surgeon has retired from the military, their age would be roughly 45–50 years and this would be a premium of about $88–144 a month [13]. Any financial planner or insurance agent will note that a lot more goes into this decision, and a good former one, will have put their clients on life insurance independent of the SGLI way before retirement. Retirement benefits continue on until the death of the service member, and this may leave the spouse with no source of income after that death. Another option for retired service members is to put part of their retirement pay into the Survivor Benefit Program (SBP). This is costly as it can be up to 55% of the monthly annuity but it does present some security for the spouse. Additionally one may opt to include children, an ex-spouse, or whomever they choose, if they do not have a spouse or child. One should consult with a financial planner with experience in military retirement to make a decision on this option. It should be noted that the default is that one will choose the SBP option, and opting out of it, requires the spouse's signature and their acknowledgement of that fact. There is also a COLA adjustment that is incorporated into the SBP and this adjusts for inflation also, but SBP probably should not replace life insurance but rather augment it [14].

When it comes to negotiating salary, one should remember that the average military surgeon will be at a different stage of life and thus accustomed to a different standard of living than the typical graduating Chief Resident or Fellow. To that end, one should have a good idea of what salary they would need to continue at least at their current living standard or to continue with their current investment strategies. Just like the military, one's pay should not be based solely on the base salary. There may be benefits like a 401 K investment plan, more pay for having a leadership position, extra monies allotted for CME, extra pay for academic pursuits (and this would likely require one to publish regularly), life insurance, and medical and dental insurance. If one were to continue the medical/dental coverage they used while in the military, they may not have need for other coverage if they have retired from Active Duty. This can be negotiated to increase the base salary. So could, too, a relocation bonus. As stated before the DOD will pay for the final relocation of their service member. The service member has up to 5 years to claim this move.

Like for any surgeon looking for a job in civilian practice, salary that is based on production can also be modified based on academic requirements and administrative position duties. As the career military surgeon may be looking for a leadership position (especially if they have been doing more administrative work for a few years), he or she may be able to negotiate a reduced production target or compensation in their salary for those duties. Most likely, the military physician will need a new state medical license. While in the military, any state license in good standing allows them to practice in a MTF. But when leaving Active Duty, that surgeon will most likely need to apply for a new one unless they plan on practicing in the state in which they currently have a license.

Finally, the surgeon should allot plenty of time to do their research (again 2 years is recommended) and put their best foot forward when applying for the new job. In most cases for the newly graduated surgeon, they will stay at their first job for 3 years before moving. For the retired military surgeon, moving again may represent additional stress as they may be looking for some stability after several moves over 20 years and because civilian practice alone will be a big change in their daily life. Going the extra mile like having one's resume professionally done, buying tailored suits for interviews, hiring a financial planner, retaining a lawyer to review the medical contract, looking at schools for their children, and estimating a prospective location's cost of living is paramount for this process, so the surgeon can find the best fit not just for their professional careers but for their family too, if that applies.

Leaving Veterans Administration or GS Employment

Leaving the GS employee or VA system will be a bit different from leaving the military, as there are less salary and benefit considerations to comprehend. Suffice it to say, though, that since the higher end salary for the most senior VA surgeons is around $355,000, it would be very difficult for someone with over 20 years in the VA system to consider leaving for financial reasons. For those with significantly less accrued time and a longer period time before they reach 25 years, they may be able to leave their GS employment and have it still make sense financially.

Overall

Government service and serving in the military can be a very rewarding experience. It won't be hard to find someone on any hospital's staff that served on Active Duty or in the VA system. There are most certainly some headaches that go along with working in the government, but the honor of serving is not something that is easily replicated. One thing that is commonly heard amongst physicians in the military or the VA system is that it is very satisfying caring for the servicemembers and veterans who have made great sacrifices for the United States. Furthermore, with more years of service, the salary of government service may not be as far from that of the civilian surgeon as it initially seems, especially if one can start collecting a pension before the age of 50 or buy a million dollar home without a down payment. Government pay will never compete with a $400,000+ salary; but, at the same time, this may require a much poorer quality of life and not much time to enjoy all of that extra money.

Disclaimer

The views expressed in this chapter are those of the authors and do not reflect the official policy of the Department of the Army, Department of Defense, or the United States Government.

References

1. Military.org. http://www.militarygme.org/. Accessed 21 Dec 2015.
2. First year physician salaries. (n.d.). http://www.valuemd.com/physician-salary-first-year.html. Accessed 22 Dec 2015.
3. General schedule (GS) locality pay area map. (n.d.). https://www.federalpay.org/gs/locality. Accessed 22 Dec 2015.
4. Annual pay ranges for physicians and dentists of the Veterans Health Administration. (2014). https://www.federalregister.gov/articles/2014/09/18/2014-22187/annual-pay-ranges-for-physicians-and-dentists-of-the-veterans-health-administration#t-7. Accessed 18 Dec 2015.
5. The Mitre Corporation report. Independent assessment of the health care delivery systems and management processes of the Department of Veterans Affairs, Volume I: integrated report. 1 Sep 15.
6. Shekelle PG. Comparison of quality of care in VA and non-VA settings: a systematic review [PDF]. Los Angeles: Evidence-based Synthesis Program (ESP) Center; 2010. http://www.hsrd.research.va.gov/publications/esp/quality.pdf.
7. Healthcare-Salaries.com. https://www.healthcare-salaries.com/physicians/general-surgeon-salary. Accessed 4 Jan 2016.

8. Federal income tax brackets for tax year 2015. (n.d.). http://www.efile.com/tax-service/tax-calculator/tax-brackets/. Accessed 15 Dec 2015.
9. FERS information eligibility. (n.d.). https://www.opm.gov/retirement-services/fers-information/eligibility. Accessed 4 Jan 2016.
10. Service CA. Compensation. (n.d.). http://www.benefits.va.gov/COMPENSATION/types-compensation.asp. Accessed 30 Nov 2015.
11. Defense Finance and Accounting Service. https://www.dfas.mil/retiredmilitary/disability/payment.html. Accessed 4 Jan 2016.
12. Education and Training. (n.d.). http://www.benefits.va.gov/gibill/post911_gibill.asp. Accessed 23 Dec 2015.
13. Hayes G. Transitioning from Military Service. (n.d.). http://www.military.com/money/retirement/military-retirement/transitioning-out-of-military-service.html. Accessed 22 Dec 2015.
14. The survivor benefit plan explained. (n.d.). http://www.military.com/benefits/survivor-benefits/the-survivor-benefit-plan-explained.html. Accessed 28 Dec 2015.

Part II

Chapter 6
Different Practice Models

Jon C. Gould

Introduction

For those reading this manual, it is unlikely you will be the one running a practice right out of training. Despite this fact, an understanding of the business side of medicine, how your performance and value is assessed, and how you can influence change in your practice is important.

Types of Practices

Although every practice situation is unique, there are two basic practice types, and a hybrid of the two can also exist. The first type of practice is supported by a third party such as a hospital, healthcare system, health maintenance organization, University, or medical school. The second type of practice is self-sufficient and unsupported (private practice). Supported practices are expected to provide services to their affiliated institution that allows this institution to make a

J.C. Gould, M.D. (✉)
Department of Surgery, Medical College of Wisconsin,
Milwaukee, WI, USA
e-mail: jgould@mcw.edu

© Springer International Publishing AG 2017   93
D.B. Renton et al. (eds.), *The SAGES Manual Transitioning to Practice*, DOI 10.1007/978-3-319-51397-3_6

profit. In exchange, the affiliated institution often covers expenses, salaries, and benefits in full or in part. Expenses may include facilities, operating expenses, and support personnel. Benefits often include salary guarantees, malpractice insurance, and health insurance. In exchange for this support, individual physicians surrender some degree of autonomy and control over their practice. This can be good or bad depending on that practice's perspective. Unsupported practices have no guarantee with regard to salary; however, there are greater opportunities to earn increased profits by controlling expenses and increasing volumes. The blended practice is essentially an unsupported practice that is partially subsidized by a third party.

In the modern era, hospitals are often paid significantly more than surgeons for the performance of a surgical procedure. As reimbursement for professional services declines and administrative needs and costs escalate, the purely unsupported model of practice is becoming less and less practical. Most remaining unsupported practices are in disciplines other than General Surgery where there is a healthy cash pay population (cosmetic or varicose vein surgery) or volume can be increased to overcome decreasing margins (LASIK surgery). Some surgeons get around these obstacles by owning the hospital outright (some orthopedic specialty hospitals, for example, or a stand-alone outpatient facility). A recent study revealed that the number of surgeons who reported to have their own self-employed practice decreased from 48 to 33% between 2001 and 2009 [1]. This decrease corresponded with an increase in the number of employed surgeons nationally. Younger surgeons and female surgeons were found to increasingly favor employment in large group practices. These employment trends were similar for both urban and rural practices. In this study, the authors conclude that factors driving these trends include the complex corporate environment, difficulties obtaining reimbursement, administrative duties, and general risks and burden of solo or small group private practices.

Where Does the Money Come from (and Where Does It Go)?

All practices must make a profit or at least cover their expenses to continue operations for any period of time. Ultimately, the success of a practice depends on the perceived quality of care provided by the practice and the ability for that practice to create and maintain a healthy referral pattern. The quality of care matters to patients, payers, and referring physicians. This is much more the case in the current era than in the past as quality measures are tracked more diligently now, and some are available to the public for review.

Surgeons and hospitals make money by providing care to patients. A unified billing system is used to generate charges based on services rendered. There are three components to this system: hospital billing, patient diagnostic coding, and patient procedural coding. Hospitals utilize the Healthcare Common Procedure Coding System (HCPCS). This is a billing system based upon Diagnosis Related Groups (DRGs). Physicians utilize diagnostic codes known as International Classification of Diseases, 10th Revision, Clinical Modification (ICD-10 CM codes). There are more than 68,000 codes in ICD-10 that describe the illness or illnesses attributable to the patient. The actual billing codes are known as the Current Procedural Terminology (CPT) codes. Reimbursement is based upon the correlation between the ICD-10 CM code and the CPT code. Modifiers may be added to the CPT codes to further explain procedures performed. A working knowledge of the coding system is important since it will impact upon patient billing and reimbursements.

Time spent with a patient is billable depending on the complexity or the time associated with the encounter. Additional billable services in a surgical practice relate to procedures performed. Consultations and history and physical exams performed on the day of a procedure are usually included in a global charge. Care provided after a procedure for a variable period of time (most often 90 days) is also included in this global charge fee. Once a service is rendered, a charge is assessed to the patient. This assessment is forwarded to a third party payer (insurance company) in most cases. With a charge generated for a service, the patient's account now has a numerical value called an "accounts receivable." Accounts receivable, or AR, means that an account is open and that any payment received can be applied against that balance. Accounts receivable is basically the amount of unpaid or outstanding bills or services. A certain percentage of these outstanding charges will not be paid. This is for reasons that might include overcharges disallowed by a third party or denied claims.

In the case of entitlement programs (Medicaid or Medicare), the overall reimbursement is based upon a complicated formula known as the Relative Value Resource Based Scale (RVRBS). RVRBS assigns procedures performed by a physician or other medical provider a relative value (measured by Relative Value Units, or RVUs) that is adjusted by geographic region (so a procedure performed in Manhattan is worth more than a procedure performed in Milwaukee). This value is then multiplied by a fixed conversion factor, which changes annually, to determine the amount of payment. Most specialties charge 200–400% of Medicare rates for their procedures and collect 40–80% of those charges after contractual adjustments and write offs. The total revenue of a practice therefore depends on the volume of care (patient encounters, but mostly surgeries), complexity of care provided (RVRBS), charges, and payer mix (percent of the practice that is entitlement programs, private insurance, HMO, etc.).

RVUs are an important concept for surgeons transitioning to practice to understand. Not only do RVUs have something to do with how much revenue your practice generates; this metric is often used to assess the productivity of individual surgeons. Depending on a surgeon's contract or incentives, RVUs may play a great role in total compensation. For each service, a payment formula contains three RVUs—one for physician work (work-related RVUs or wRVU), one for practice expense, and one for malpractice expense. On average, the proportion of costs for Medicare is 52%, 44%, and 4%, respectively. Historically, a private group of 29 (mostly specialist) physicians—the American Medical Association's Specialty Society Relative Value Scale Update Committee (RUC)—have largely determined Medicare's RVU physician work values. These three RVUs are combined to form what are known as total RVUs.

The RVUs for procedures typically performed by General Surgeons can vary widely. Although used as a metric of productivity or clinical work, in certain specialties and for certain common procedure this correlation is poor [2, 3]. Surgeons should familiarize themselves with the RVUs associated with the procedures they perform most commonly. Published benchmarks for RVUs by specialty are available and are often used to set productivity goals. The most commonly used benchmarks for General Surgeons are the University Health Consortium (UHC) and Medical Group Management Association (MGMA) benchmarks. These benchmarks can differ significantly (by more than 1000 RVUs). In an academic practice, activities such as teaching and research may be expected. Depending on the magnitude of the role or contribution expected, these RVU benchmarks may become unrealistic for academic surgeons devoting a significant portion of their time to activities that don't generate RVUs. A surgical residency program director or a faculty member with a basic science lab should not be expected to succeed at these academic endeavors and still meet the RVU benchmark established by a 100% clinical effort surgeon. In an academic practice setting, these "nonclinical" activities need to be funded. Medical Schools and Universities may provide funds to Departments or individual surgeons to offset the lost clinical productivity associated with these important missions. Researchers may be provided with startup funds from a variety of sources with the understanding that their research will need to be funded by other sources after a certain period of time (extramural grants). A typical academic practice funds a large part of the education and research mission with dollars generated through clinical work. In these settings, each provider is considered 1.0 FTE (Full Time Equivalent), and their work will be defined by the amount of time they spend on clinical work, and the time they spend on research/teaching. For example, the program director mentioned above may be 0.6 FTE clinical, and 0.4 FTE administrative. His RVU goal will be modified by the 0.6 FTE that is his clinical practice. Most surgical departments are therefore composed of a mix of surgeons who devote various portions of their effort to these different activities. Due in part to this fact, academic surgeon salaries (at least for early career academic surgeons) tends to be less than those of private practice surgeons.

A major expense of any practice is physician salaries. Providing surgeons with compensation in line with their fair market value is important when it comes to successful recruitment, retention, and satisfaction. Salaries for surgeons are set based on many factors. The MGMA publishes benchmarks for both private practice and academic surgeons with adjustments for tenure, role, and responsibility. Individual surgeon contracts are discussed in another chapter in this manual. Total compensation for a surgeon can be set at a fixed value or based on productivity or other factors.

How Is Physician Performance Assessed?

More and more in this era of transparency, public reporting of hospital and physician performance, and value-based care, physicians are being evaluated and leaders are being held accountable for performance metrics in addition to RVUs. The Institute of Medicine defines "Aims for Improvement" across six domains of healthcare quality: safety, effectiveness, timeliness, efficiency, patient-centeredness, and equity. The Center for Medicare and Medicaid Services (CMS) is withholding a certain percent of payments for services rendered based on performance in these, and other domains. Payers are aligning with healthcare systems that demonstrate quality (including efficiency or cost) and driving patients to these organizations. Individual physicians are being held accountable for quality metrics like never before. Readmission rates, patient satisfaction, and even costs for particular procedures are metrics used to assess performance. Running a surgical practice is now very much about understanding these different quality metrics, how they are assessed, and how the practice and individual surgeons are performing in these areas. These topics will be covered in much more detail in another chapter of this manual.

Depending on the mission of the organization and the practice itself, performance may be assessed in other ways. A surgeon with a major role in education may be measured based on his/her teaching evaluations, number of curricula developed, or even publications in the education domain. A surgeon with a significant research commitment will be evaluated based on grants attained and extramural funding as well as publications and impact. For those running a practice with faculty spending time and effort on these activities, it is important to communicate what is expected and how performance will be assessed. Finally, service to the practice or the affiliated institution is also important. Surgeons may be expected to serve on institutional or department committees and task forces. When it comes time for a promotion in an academic position (Assistant to Associate Professor for example), clinical excellence, research, teaching, and service are the four domains often taken into account when assessing the merit of a proposed promotion. If you are on an academic track, you should review your institution's criteria for promotion early in your tenure.

Leadership

Let's close this chapter with a word about leadership. Leadership is obviously important when running a practice. Even fresh out of residency or fellowship, leadership skills are called for and of great importance. We are all leaders in different contexts, and failure of junior faculty to recognize this can slow down their development and limit their potential. There are many conceptual frameworks of what it takes to be a leader. There is no one right theory or approach.

Leadership in surgery entails professionalism, technical competence, motivation, innovation, teamwork, communication skills, decision-making, business acumen, emotional competence, resilience, and effective teaching. Leadership skills can be developed through experience, observation, and education using a framework including mentoring, coaching, networking, stretch assignments, action learning, and feedback [4].

The personality and style of any leader has a significant impact on the culture of a team, organization, or a surgical practice. There is no ideal style, but there are personality traits that characterize effective leaders and styles that suit some teams or environments more than others. Styles can range from democratic to autocratic. Good leaders know how to adapt to the situation and people they are leading. This is as true for surgeons as for any other professional occupation.

In their book, the Leadership Challenge [5], Kouzes and Posner outline the ten commitments of leadership, paraphrased here. Leaders need to find their voice by clarifying personal values. They set the example by aligning actions and shared values. They envision the future (their goals short and long term) and enlist others in a common vision by appealing to shared aspirations. They search for opportunities, generate small wins, and learn from their mistakes (there will be plenty). They foster collaboration and strengthen others by empowering them. They recognize contributions by showing appreciation and creating a spirit of community. It is important for leaders to remember that an effective team can accomplish far more than a group of individuals.

Surgeons must both lead and manage. Leadership means a focus on setting direction, motivating others, and ensuring that the operational elements are safely and efficiently delivered. Managing tends to involve a focus on processes, systems, plans, and schedules and ensuring that these work effectively and objectives are achieved. The boundaries between leading and managing have become increasingly blurred and in practice the roles overlap.

There are a multitude of leadership books and courses sponsored by organizations such as SAGES and the American College of Surgeons. Young surgeons, especially those who are asked to take on meaningful leadership positions, should invest in their own personal and professional development by spending time on these activities.

Part of being a good leader is personal effectiveness and focus. In his book, Good to Great [6], Jim Collins discusses the parable of the fox and the hedgehog. In his famous essay, "The Hedgehog and the Fox," Isaiah Berlin divided the world into hedgehogs and foxes, based upon an ancient Greek parable: "The fox knows many things, but the hedgehog knows one big thing." While Collins' focus is on companies that made the leap from good to great, the Hedgehog Concept can apply to surgeons as well. The concept is simple and based on a deep understanding about the answers to the following three questions:

What you can be the best in the world at (and, equally important, what you cannot be the best in the world at).

What drives your economic (academic, clinical, etc.) engine?

What are you deeply passionate about?

The good-to-great companies focused on those activities that ignited their passion. The idea here is not to stimulate passion but to discover what makes you passionate.

Aligning your passion, expertise, and effort in the same direction makes you a more effective person. Understanding what direction you are headed in helps you focus on the activities that will get you there, and even to say no to activities that will distract you from this mission. Saying no to the wrong opportunity is one of the hardest things a young surgeon needs to learn how to do.

Conclusions

Running a surgical practice is a major responsibility that calls for in-depth knowledge of healthcare finance, program development, mentorship, team building, decision-making, and effective communication skills. The knowledge and skill set needed is acquired through a combination of experience, observation, mentorship, and education that may include courses offered locally, through universities, or by professional societies. The development of these skills and fostering of the necessary knowledge is a gradual process that begins very early in a surgeon's career.

References

1. Charles AG, Ortiz-Pujols S, Ricketts T, et al. The employed surgeon: a changing professional paradigm. JAMA Surg. 2013;148(4): 323–8.
2. Shah DR, Bold RJ, Yang AD, et al. Relative value units poorly correlate with measures of surgical effort and complexity. J Surg Res. 2014;190(2):465–70.
3. Schwartz DA, Hui X, Velopulos CG, et al. Does relative value unit-based compensation shortchange the acute care surgeon? J Trauma Acute Care Surg. 2014;76(1):84–92.
4. Patel VM, Warren O, Humphris P, et al. What does leadership in surgery entail? ANZ J Surg. 2010;80(12):876–83.
5. Kouzes JM, Posner BZ. The leadership challenge. 4th ed. San Francisco: Jossey-Bas; 2007.
6. Collins J. Good to great. 1st ed. New York: Harper business; 2001.

Chapter 7
How Do I Grow a Practice: Marketing, Word of Mouth, Getting Referrals

Valerie Halpin

Building a Practice Starts with Service Excellence

The first step to growing a successful practice is the physician accepting responsibility for service excellence. The physician sets the tone for how the practice is run with leadership by example. This means treating not just patients with care and expertise, but also your staff and other physicians. Take the time to get to know your staff by name both in the office and the hospital. Greet them with a pleasant hello when you enter the room. This will go a long way to building collaborative relationships with patients and other healthcare professionals. It cannot be stressed enough that the way you treat the people around you will reflect on you, and determine how they treat you. The classic axiom of the successful General Surgeon is: Affable, Available, and Able. Service excellence meshes well with this axiom.

V. Halpin, M.D. (✉)
Weight and Diabetes Institute, Legacy Good Samaritan Hospital, 1040 NW 22nd Avenue, Portland, OR 97209, USA
e-mail: vhalpin@lhs.org

© Springer International Publishing AG 2017
D.B. Renton et al. (eds.), *The SAGES Manual Transitioning to Practice*, DOI 10.1007/978-3-319-51397-3_7

Building Referral Sources

Where do patients come from? The first step is identifying where referrals come from. Depending on your specialty, referrals may come from returning patients, friends, and family of your previous patients, other physicians, taking call, or direct to consumer marketing. Each one of these areas requires a different strategy to develop the referral source.

Referrals from Other Patients

This is an area that will take time. You have to take care of a few patients before any will send you their friends and family. Make sure it is clearly posted in your office that you are accepting new patients. How you take care of your patients really matters and will determine if they will keep coming back or send someone else to you. To achieve this, tools like **AIDET** can be used by you and your staff. **AIDET** is an acronym for five communication behaviors used to achieve patient satisfaction. Patients and their families have a lot of anxiety when they are accessing healthcare and this can help manage it. **AIDET** stands for:

Acknowledge patients by their name and with a smile at every encounter.

Introduce yourself to patients by your name and what your role is. You may think you do not need to identify yourself as the surgeon, but patients see so many people when they are in the healthcare setting, that it may not be obvious to them what your role is. This is true in both the office and the hospital settings.

Keep patients informed of the **duration** of the encounter. In the office, your staff should let patients know if you will be delayed and give them the option of rescheduling if a delay does not work for them. In the hospital, you can let families know what is the expected time a case may take and when you will be speaking with them afterwards. Keep them informed of how they will be notified of delays. When you speak with the family following surgery, let them know what the expected time in recovery will be and when and where they can expect to see their family member again.

Provide a clear **explanation** of what you are going to do during the encounter. In an office visit, this could be a simple explanation such as "I'm going to ask you some questions about your medical history to learn more about why you are here and do a physical exam. When we are done with that part we can discuss what additional testing we need to do, and then treatment options."

Finally, say **thank you**. You can thank patients for the opportunity and privilege of caring for them. If you are running late, thank them for waiting. This helps build a relationship of mutual respect and demonstrates your understanding that their time is valuable too.

Germane to a surgery practice are a few more rules that can be added.

Responding to patient calls. Have a mechanism of returning phone calls in a timely and professional manner. In the beginning when you are not busy, do it yourself. Consider calling all of your patients personally a few days after outpatient procedures or after hospital discharges. This will go a long way to set yourself apart from other providers. Once you have established a strong reputation you do not necessarily have to do this for all patients yourself, you can have a delegate do it. It is helpful to continue to do so with your most difficult patients, or patients who seem to be calling your office a lot. You can often provide much greater reassurance to your patients than anyone else on your staff can. Reassurance is the most common thing that patients need when they call the office after procedures.

Schedule realistically. Be honest about scheduling your cases and clinics. Don't overextend yourself. A case that took you 1 h in residency may take you two or more when you first start out on your own. You may be in a new facility with a new assistant, new OR staff, and new instrumentation. All the members of your team (including yourself) will need time to learn your routines. Review your operative schedule weekly with your scheduler. Schedulers often do not understand the nuances of cases. You cannot rely on them to schedule cases for the correct amount of time until you have adequately trained them.

Transitioning to a new practice will also lengthen the amount of time it takes you to get your other work done including rounding and communicating with consultants. Plan that extra time into your schedule. Everyone around you will respect you more for being able to accurately plan your (and therefore their) time.

Clinic visits may also take longer when you are first getting started. Allow for a ramp up period. As more and more practices are utilizing electronic health records, allow some additional time to build and refine templates and order sets.

Finally, if you have family responsibilities, allow some cushion in your professional schedule so you can meet them. Don't plan your work schedule so that you will be down to the last wire to get your child from daycare on time.

Referrals from Other Doctors AKA "Relationship Building"

Identify existing relationships. What are the preexisting referral patterns to your practice? Will some of those patients be distributed to you? How will that be decided? Are you hospital employed with a big primary care or medical subspecialty base? Learn about recommended referral patterns within your organization. Make sure that you are included in any queues that distribute referrals in your specialty. In the age of electronic health records, take the time to make sure that your contact information is available and accurate.

Build relationships with referring physicians. Whether you are starting in an established group of the same specialty or you are new specialty type within your practice it is important to build relationships. Take the time to **meet the physicians** in your region that could refer to you. Large practices and hospital systems have outreach personnel to help schedule meet and greets with referring physicians. Identify that person and get started. Participate in social/professional activities such as town hall meetings or your local medical or surgical society if available. Go where other doctors go. If there is a doctor's dining area in your hospital, eat there. Introduce yourself. Learn about the other providers there and learn their needs so that you can identify yourself as a possible solution.

Make it easy for them to refer patients to you. Don't make them do all the work. If they have talked to you personally, offer to take it from there and either make the appointment or call the patient yourself. Make sure your office staff are well educated on the referral process and the scope of your practice. Once you have seen a patient, respond back to the referring physician quickly in the form of a copy of your note or a consultation letter that is clear and well written. Get back to the referring provider before your patient does. The fastest way depends on your local practice environment. Electronic health records can be immediate. Learn what your referring provider prefers. Sometimes email and fax are still the fastest options. If you have a complicated patient, communicate directly with their other medical providers, in particular regarding areas of conflicting management. While electronic communication is efficient and easy, some complicated conversations are better had over the telephone or in person. Consider calling referring physicians after you have operated on one of their patients, in particular those patients who will need ongoing follow up from that physician. If you use consultants or hospitalist services in the hospital, communicate frequently with the other providers. This will help to minimize miscommunications and improve patient care, as well as build your relationship with other physicians.

Be available and accessible. Be willing to see new patients at the convenience of the patient and the referring physician. Offer to see patients same day or on days you are not normally in the clinic if it is urgent. Give the referring physician your email and cell phone number. Answer your cell phone when called.

Establish yourself as an expert. Determine what types of patients you want to see. Provide educational talks on your specialty at local grand rounds, at regional or state society meetings, clinic administrative meetings, CME events, quality meetings, etc. Build a schedule that allows you to see those types of patients quickly. When you start doing a new innovative technique or even just something new to your practice, send out a letter to referring physicians identifying the new service.

Be willing to take some of the both difficult and bread and butter cases. This will go a long way to establishing loyalty from your referring providers. They really don't like it if they've sent you a lot of good cases and then you refuse to take a lesser case. Take care of them with the same level of attention that you would a more ideal case.

Send patients back. Some doctors may not like to send patients to you if they end up losing the patient all together. Make sure you send patients back to referring physicians and take the time to make sure they know that you have. If you identify other health maintenance needs such as colonoscopy, mammograms, and diabetes exams, send them back to their referring primary physician.

Taking Call

Plan to take call for your specialty at your hospital. This can help provide you with new patients until your elective practice is up and running. It also builds good will within your local medical community. Find out who makes the schedule and how calls are assigned. Is it part of a medical staff requirement or your contract or is it voluntary? Take your share. Try to align your call responsibilities to fit in well with your elective practice. For example, if you are taking call at a busy hospital, don't take call the night before your clinic and then have to cancel your clinic for an emergency case. If you are proactive in signing up for call, you can potentially get the shifts that work for you, rather than shifts that compromise your ability to meet your other professional and personal obligations.

Direct to Consumer Marketing

The two most important steps in marketing are to do your research and to make a plan. Determine what types of patients you are trying to market to. Establish your digital presence online. Find out from your practice management what online marketing materials already exist. Make sure you are added to all websites and social media sites with a professional photograph. Encourage your happy patients to fill out online reviews. Promptly respond to any negative online reviews taking care to acknowledge any concerns and present a plan for improvement. Some specialties can purchase services that generate a periodic electronic newsletter where you can brand it with your practice, but you do not have to develop all the content. This is a way to keep reminding patients about you. Participate in community health fairs or events.

There are many other more expensive resources such as local and national consulting agencies, as well as television, radio, and print ads. These are great if you have a lot of financial resources, but not necessary if you can build on all the other elements discussed above.

Tracking Referral Sources

Establish a way to track your referral sources. You should discuss this with your practice administrator. If you are in an integrated health system with electronic referrals, there may be a report that is automatically generated for each practice with electronic referrals. If you don't have this capability and for patients that are not referred in this manner, there are any number of ways to obtain the information. Your office staff can ask patients when they call to make an appointment or when registering them at their first appointment. It can also be a simple check box on your registration questionnaire. You can purchase online and mobile services available that can streamline this process for you. Once you have this data, use it to your benefit. Has a certain physician stopped referring your patients? Find out why. Are you receiving more referrals from one physician, make sure you send them a letter thanking them for the referrals.

Schedule practice building into your weekly routine. It requires your attention to ensure it is a priority with your staff. Make sure this is a regular agenda item at your administrative meetings. Allow time in your schedule to do the activities that you will need to do to build the type of practice you want.

Prioritize your Referral Base

Make sure you take care of the physicians who do refer your patients. This means going the extra mile when it is not always convenient. Make sure you can get their patients in quickly. Be good to their staff. It is often office staff who actually do the referrals. When you call to talk to other physicians, be courteous and kind to their staff. Show off your charming personality and great bedside manner. If you are rude to them, they will not forget it.

Referral Rewards

Incentivize patients who refer others back to you. This can be something as simple as a handwritten thank you note or coffee cards, on up to discounting out of pocket elective procedures. You can also send them information on something that may be of interest to them such as information on a new medical treatment or procedure.

Summary

Growing a practice is based on strong physician leadership and service excellence with focus on building relationships, being responsive and available. The one part of the axiom

Affable, Available, and Able that was not touched on was ABLE. Your greatest source of continued referrals from patients, their friends, and other physicians are good outcomes for your surgical patients. If you are just starting out and have a difficult case scheduled, make sure you have help available if needed. Don't put yourself on an island. Nothing can stall a career faster when getting started than a string of complications to your first patients.

Bibliography

1. D.A. Popowich. Reputation, reliability, and responsiveness. Building and maintaining a referral base. SAGES 2015
2. 11 Secrets to doubling doctor referrals to your hospital or practice. Healthcare Success Strategies. c 2012

Chapter 8
Retirement: 401k, Roth IRAs, College Funds, and More

David S. Strosberg, Sara E. Martin del Campo, and David B. Renton

Introduction

THE CASE TO BE MADE: Transitioning away from a surgical practice to retirement requires advanced planning and discussion with family, friends, peers, and professional advisors. It is well recognized that many general surgeons continue to practice beyond the customary retirement age of 65. The most common reason for a surgeon to continue practicing is a personal fulfillment in one's career. However, while

D.S. Strosberg, M.D.
Department of Surgery, The Ohio State University Wexner
Medical Center, 410 W 10th Ave # N717,
Columbus, OH 43205, USA

S.E. Martin del Campo, M.D., M.S.
Department of Surgery, The Ohio State University Wexner Medical
Center, 410 W 10th Ave # N717, Columbus, OH 43205, USA

Center for Minimally Invasive Surgery, The Ohio State
University Wexner Medical Center, Columbus, OH, USA

D.B. Renton, M.D., M.S.P.H., F.A.C.S. (✉)
Department of Surgery, The Ohio State University Wexner
Medical Center, 410 W 10th Ave # N717,
Columbus, OH 43205, USA

Center for Minimally Invasive Surgery, The Ohio State
University Wexner Medical Center, Columbus, OH, USA
e-mail: david.renton@osumc.edu

© Springer International Publishing AG 2017   113
D.B. Renton et al. (eds.), *The SAGES Manual Transitioning
to Practice*, DOI 10.1007/978-3-319-51397-3_8

some surgeons do not fully retire at age 65, many that remain in their practice will reduce their operative volume after age 60 [1]. Approximately 17% of practicing surgeons continue to operate after 70 years of age according to a 1994 survey. It is also important to remember that the average surgeon does not begin his or her career until the age of 31. This is 10 years after the average college graduate begins their career and an important consideration in planning for future retirement. Another consideration in continuing to practice may be the need or desire to continue one's income. In the following discussion, financial retirement preparation issues are addressed so that a surgeon is financially prepared for retirement whether or not he or she chooses to leave or reduce their operative volumes at or near retirement age.

ASSEMBLE AN ADVISORY TEAM: Albert Einstein, the German-born twentieth century theoretical physicist is quoted as saying "Out of clutter, find simplicity." Financial retirement preparation needs to be made simple, out of what may appear cluttered. We would add that to find simplicity in the clutter, a surgeon needs to be deliberate in his or her retirement preparation. The surgeon is best served if the deliberate preparation for retirement is best addressed and implemented early in a surgeon's career to provide flexibility in approaches and efficiency in asset accumulation. The preparation process can be referred to as "Financial Planning." Financial Planning requires analysis and implementation coordinating several areas of expertise, including legal, tax, insurance, retirement plan design, and investment advice. Because Financial Planning is a multifaceted approach, surgeons may want to develop a team of experts to guide him or her through one's clinical career. To coordinate these specialists, a primary advisor having a broad understanding of a surgeon's financial objectives is important. Primary advisors may be found with a plethora of backgrounds including, legal, accounting, tax, and financial planning. While an individual advisor's area of expertise has some bearing on the selection decision, of paramount importance is the individual's experience, coordinating capabilities, personality, and communication skills.

DETERMINE THE FINANCIAL TARGET: When fully or partially leaving the workforce, income replacement may come from one or more of four primary sources: (1) savings, including retirement accounts; (2) annuities; (3) permanent insurance policies; and, (4) social security benefits. While each of these sources has benefits and risk, a surgeon must initially estimate future financial goals. One obvious goal is an estimate of income needs of the surgeon when he or she retires. Additionally, future goals may include gifts and bequests to family and charity. To determine this amount, a practical way to describe these desires is to state the amounts in today's dollars, i.e., the present value of the goal. With the goal stated in today's dollars, the surgeon's Financial Planning team will need to address how many dollars it will take to accomplish the goal(s) at the future retirement date, taking into account inflation, taxes, and investment return estimates. The resulting analysis will be probabilistic rather than definitive. Therefore, the planning process needs to be updated periodically to assure the surgeon that the asset accumulation is on plan to meet the goal(s).

For the typical American, many financial analysts recommend a total savings sufficient for a 4% withdrawal rate of saving assets to produce 70% of one's annual salary. This withdrawal rate historically preserves asset value over time, assuming investments allocated in approximately 50% in stocks and 50% bonds. Using this calculation, a surgeon with a $200,000 annual salary should anticipate having a total savings of $5,000,000 at the start of retirement, which may be significantly more than what is needed. While analysts assume that a retiree will require 70% of preretirement income, the actual number may be considerably lower for high-income earners because expenses in retirement may be significantly reduced, i.e., mortgages paid off, life insurance premiums fully funded and children's education costs funded. The United States Department of Labor Lifetime Income Calculator (http://www.askebsa.dol.gov/lia/home) may be a useful tool, in addition to a surgeon's Financial Planning Team, to estimate monthly lifetime income based on the individual's current account balance and projected value of that account balance at age 65, factoring in investment returns of 7% and inflation rates of 3% annually [2].

ATTAINING THE FINANCIAL TARGET: Albert Einstein is quoted as saying that, "Compound interest is the eighth wonder of the world. He who understands it, earns it ... he who doesn't ... pays it." In other words, a dollar efficiently saved today allows for compounded growth toward the financial resources to support financial retirement needs. For example, saving 10% of pre-tax income of $250,000 for 25 years compared to 20 years with a starting $0 account balance will yield a $315,661 greater total account balance, and a $1638 higher income per month (Fig. 8.1). When planning for retirement, establishing a plan to accumulate retirement assets is important to begin early in the surgeon's career. If not established early in a career, establishing a financial plan for retirement becomes even more critical if retirement goals are to be met.

The following accumulation methods have been organized into income benefits and asset accumulation benefits. While neither exhaustive nor detailed, it should provide a framework for a surgeon's understanding and communication with his or her Financial Planning Team.

	Scenario 1	Scenario 2	Difference	
Retirement Age (years)	65	65	0	
Current Account Balance ($)	0	0	0	
Current Annual Contribution ($)	25,000	25,000	0	
Age at Start of Savings (years)	45	40	**5**	
Projected Account Balance ($)	815,262	1,130,923	**315,661**	
Lifetime Income Per Month ($)	4,231	5,869	**1,638**	

*Source- United States Department of Labor Lifetime Income Calculator

Fig. 8.1 Lifetime income calculations (asterisk)—a comparison of 5 years difference of savings

Income Benefits, Social Security: Social Security is the US national pension program for Americans who pay into the program while employed [3]. It will not cover all expenses while retired; rather, it should be used as a supplement. The calculation for an individual's benefit is complex and is based on the number of years worked and paid into Social Security and average national wage. Formulas are applied so that high-income earners will receive disproportionately less than low-income earners. The earliest age of eligibility is 62 years, at which time the individual will receive 70% of the full benefit amount. Full retirement age is 67 years in order to receive 100% of benefits. Each year of delaying benefits provides an 8% increase in income up to age 70 (124% of primary insurance amount). In addition, Social Security is taxable based on the benefit amount. A physician with a $250,000 annual salary may expect to receive $20,000–$40,000 in benefits annually. The Social Security Administration provides several online calculators that may assist with your financial planning, including the Retirement Calculator that estimates your monthly benefits based on your actual Social Security earnings record (https://www.ssa.gov/planners/benefitcalculators.html).

Income Benefits, Pension Plans: Pension plans are retirement accounts that are arranged and managed by the employer. While pension plans are "sister" retirement programs to contributory plans including 401 k, profit sharing plans, and simplified employee plans, pension plans are designed to provide retirement income whereas defined contribution plans are designed to provide a pre-tax savings vehicle providing an asset for retirement that will generate an unspecified and nonguaranteed amount of income However, a *defined-benefit*, including a cash balance pension plan, guarantees a certain payout amount at retirement according to a fixed formula, usually considering salary and the number of years of membership in the plan. It is important to recognize career opportunities that may have a lower pre-tax compensation with favorable pension plans, including state and federal retirement systems, as this may have a greater contribution to one's retirement income.

Income Benefits, Annuities: Annuities are another tax-deferred investment option which allows one to invest money and then select for payments to be withdrawn at a future date. The income can be distributed monthly, quarterly, annually, or in the form of a lump sum. A fixed annuity is one managed by an investment company and provides a guaranteed payout; whereas a variable annuity has a payout determined by the performance of the underlying investment and is managed by the individual. In addition, one can opt for a deferred annuity, in which money is invested for a period of time until one is ready for withdrawals (typically in retirement) or an immediate annuity, which allows for withdrawals shortly after making the initial investment. Annuities are purchased with after-tax dollars and have no contribution limits. They have commission and other fees which, in the aggregate, are higher than many other retirement investments.

Asset Accumulation, Savings Accounts: Investment portfolios should comprise both short-term and long-term investments. Short-term investments include savings, certificates of deposit, and short-term bonds; while long-term investments include longer term bonds, variable annuities, and stocks. Income during retirement may be divided in three main categories: taxable, tax-free, and tax-deferred. *Taxable income* includes those accounts outside of structured retirement savings plans, such as traditional savings accounts, stocks, mutual funds, and real estate. Taxable income does not offer a tax-benefit at any time to the individual. *Tax-free income* refers to funds that were invested with after-tax money and may be withdrawn at retirement age free of any additional taxation. Examples of tax-free investments include Roth Individual Retirement Accounts (IRAs), life insurance, and bonds. *Tax-deferred income* uses pre-tax funds, which may be withdrawn at retirement. However, all money withdrawn is taxed at the standard income tax rates. Examples of tax-deferred income include traditional IRAs, 401(k) and 403(b), 457 deferred compensation plans, and annuities. This offers the advantage of pre-tax payroll deduction, company matching, and choices for investment. Experts recommend maximizing contributions into tax-free and tax-deferred accounts and then use taxable income accounts as a supplement to those investments. There are specific rules set out by the Internal Revenue Service regarding the distribution of retirement plans. If money is withdrawn from a retirement plan before the age of 59.5 years, there are considerable penalties. However, there are harsher penalties if the required amount is not withdrawn before 70.5 years as well. In addition, a beneficiary should be named to reduce tax implications at the time of one's death.

401(k), 403(b), and 457 Company Plans

The 401(k) plan, named for its respective section of the Internal Revenue Code, allows employees to invest a portion of their paycheck before taxes are taken out through payroll deductions [4]. In this example of tax-deferred income, the savings can multiply tax-free until retirement, at which point the entire withdrawal will be taxed as income. One of the major benefits of this plan is tax deduction; funds are pre-tax and are therefore tax deductible. This offers an attractive benefit for high-income earners to reduce annual taxes and potentially decrease their tax bracket. Although limits are set by the Internal Revenue Code, IRS regulations and the Department of Labor, the annual contribution limit at this writing is $17,500 in 2014, increasing to $18,000 in 2015 (with an additional $5500 in 2014 and $6000 in 2015 if the employee is age 50 or older). The funds contributed to the 401(k) are then invested with the 401(k) provider. Many employers will then match an employee's contribution. Employer contributions do not count against the individual contribution limits, but do count against the total 401(k) contribution limit-currently $52,000 in 2014. In using a 401(k) plan, it is important to identify one's savings goal; if the employer contributes 3%, the individual may need to increase his or her contribution to 12% to match a 15% goal.

Most financial analysts recommend increasing the individual's contribution to the employer match. A 403(b) plan is similar to a 401(k) plan except that 403(b) plan is only available to employees of tax-exempt organizations. A 457 plan is available to state and local public employees as well as some nonprofit organizations. It is also similar to the 401(k) and 403(b) plans but without a penalty for early withdrawals though one would still owe the income tax on the money withdrawn early [5].

Traditional IRA: A Traditional IRA is tax-deferred retirement savings account that comes in either a tax-deductible or tax-nondeductible form. A deductible IRA allows the investor to deduct the contributions on annual taxes, whereas a nondeductible IRA is funded with after-tax dollars. However, only those without an employer retirement plan or with an income less than $89,000 for a married couple or $56,000 for an individual can qualify for a deductible IRA. Amounts in your traditional IRA including earnings and gains are taxed at the time of distribution.

Roth IRAs

A Roth IRA is a popular example of tax-free income. Roth IRAs use after-tax funds to be placed in favorable retirement savings accounts, which can be withdrawn without tax after 5 years beginning at age 59½. For years 2013–2016, the maximum amount that can be contributed to a Roth IRA is $5500 for those age 49 and below, and $6500 for those age 50 and above. *However high-income earners may not be eligible.* For 2016, single filers earning up to $117,000 can qualify for a full contribution or up to $132,000 for a partial contribution. Married filers earning up to $184,000 qualify for a full contribution, or up to $194,000 for a partial contribution. Those who are married and filing separately can only contribute if the investing spouse's income is less than $10,000.

Life Insurance Retirement Plan

A Life Insurance Retirement Plan (LIRP) mimics many of the characteristics of a Roth IRA, without the income limitations, allowing high-income individuals to participate. The investor purchases a cash-value life insurance policy that is overfunded for at least 10 years. There are no contribution caps, but contributions into the policy are not tax deductible. Once the value of the deposits approaches the cash value of the policy, usually after approximately 15 years, tax-free loans or withdrawals can then be made from the policy to supplement retirement income. Death benefits paid to beneficiaries are also income tax-free. However, if the life insurance policy lapses, all distributions become immediately taxable. In addition, policies must be carefully structured, and the LIRP offers the greatest advantage to investors who have already maximized other tax-advantage retirement savings plans.

Investment Allocation, Long-term returns, short-term volatility, and implementation vehicles: To reach a surgeon's retirement goals, the Financial Planning Team should among other things, establish an investment allocation based on qualitative and quantitative measures. Qualitative considerations should include the surgeon's risk tolerance, i.e., acceptance of short-term depreciation for long-term appreciation. Quantitative measures analyze various investment assets for their risk, return, and correlation of these variables to one another.

Investment asset classes are groupings of various investments that have similarity in structure, volatility, and returns. Two of the asset classes typically utilized by surgeons are stocks and bonds. For this discussion, more specialized asset classes such as precious metals, private equity, real estate, and hedge funds are not summarized.

Stocks: A stock is an ownership share of a company. Money is made off of stocks when a stock goes up in value as more people are interested in purchasing it. The owner of the stock only makes money when the stock is then sold at a higher price than it was purchased. Companies may also issue dividends, which are payouts to the stockholders reflecting the company's earnings. Historically, stocks have produced larger long-term gains than other asset classes, at an average of 9.8% per year since 1926, but they carry more short-term risk due to variability in the market. Stocks that are purchased outside of tax-free or tax-deferred retirement accounts are taxed annually. Dividends and any profits made on a sale of stock are taxed up to a rate of 15%.

Bonds: Investing in bonds is another method of securing income in retirement. In purchasing a bond, the investor is loaning out money to the issuer for a certain period of time. In return, the investor gets the loan back in addition to a fixed interest rate on the loan at the specified maturity date. Bonds provide some advantages in that they are generally more stable than stocks, they pay interest regularly, allowing for a predictable amount of income, and the income is tax-free on many lower-yield government bonds. However, bonds are subject to income loss should the issuer be unable to make its payment, and the fixed interest rate may not keep up with inflation across the time of maturation.

Mutual funds: Mutual funds are not, in themselves, an asset class. Rather, mutual funds are a pooling method of many thousands of investors with a common investment strategy. Mutual funds can invest in stocks, bonds, and other asset classes. The decision of what to buy or sell is determined by professional fund managers based on strategy outlined in the prospectus of the fund. The advantage of these funds is that they provide broader diversification for risk reduction in investing, with a lower management fee.

Exchange Traded Funds: While most mutual funds are actively managed, i.e., an investment manager selects the securities, a passive pooling fund that generally invests in indexes rather than selecting specific securities, is known as an exchange traded fund.

Conclusion: Retirement presents new and often underappreciated emotional, psychological, and financial hurdles.

Preparation by developing new interests and fulfilling hobbies is essential in retirement planning. But in addition to that, retirement requires careful financial planning to maintain an acceptable quality of life. An individual must consider their postretirement expenses and the use of multiple retirement savings plans to prepare. In addition to personal career fulfillment, prolonging the length of time until withdrawing retirement funds can have significant financial benefits, so the earlier you start the better off you will be. We strongly recommend consulting with professional financial experts throughout one's clinical practice to plan accordingly for your retirement needs.

References

1. Williams TE Jr, Ellison EC (2008) Population analysis predicts a future critical shortage of general surgeons. Surgery 144(4):548–554, discussion 554–546
2. United States Department of Labor Lifetime Income Calculator. Benefits planner: your future benefits. http://www.askebsa.dol.gov/lia/home. Accessed Oct 2016
3. Social Security: official social security website. http://www.ssa.gov/planners/index.html. Accessed Oct 2016
4. Internal Revenue Service, United States Department of the Treasury. Tax topics—Topic 424 – 401(k) plans. http://www.irs.gov/taxtopics/tc424.html. Accessed Oct 2016
5. Internal Revenue Service, United States Department of the Treasury. Types of retirement plans. http://www.irs.gov/Retirement-Plans/Plan-Sponsor/Types-of-Retirement-Plans-1. Accessed Oct 2016

Chapter 9
Surgical Quality and Safety: Current Initiatives and Future Directions

Michelle C. Nguyen and Susan D. Moffatt-Bruce

Key Points

- Despite improved therapies and technology, preventable medical errors and adverse events in surgery continue to occur.
- Error can be classified into four groups: diagnostic, treatment, preventative, or other errors.
- Several initiatives have been implemented to improve patient safety: (1) Patient Safety and Quality Improvement Act, (2) Medicare Prescription Drug, Improvement, and Modernization Act, and (3) Bundled Payments for Care Improvement Initiative.
- Pressures for improving value-based care have led to the linkage of quality to reimbursements implemented by the Hospital Readmissions Reduction

(continued)

M.C. Nguyen, M.D. • S.D. Moffatt-Bruce, M.D., Ph.D., F.A.C.S. (✉)
Department of General Surgery, The Ohio State University
Wexner Medical Center, Columbus, OH, USA, 43221

Division of Thoracic Surgery, The Ohio State University
Wexner Medical Center, Columbus, OH, USA, 43221
e-mail: Susan.Moffatt-Bruce@osumc.edu

© Springer International Publishing AG 2017   125
D.B. Renton et al. (eds.), *The SAGES Manual Transitioning to Practice*, DOI 10.1007/978-3-319-51397-3_9

(continued)

> Program, Hospital Value-Based Purchasing Program, and the Hospital-Acquired Condition Program.
> - Established quality improvement programs such as the Agency for Healthcare and Research Quality, The American College of Surgeons National Surgical Quality Improvement Program, and University HealthSystem Consortium provide risk-adjusted quality data to participating hospitals to benchmark performance.
> - Human error is inevitable, but defective systems can be fixed to detect and prevent errors. The use of Crew Resource Management and Surgical Checklists are methods to reduce systemic error
> - Resident duty hours and physician burnout can impact patient safety and quality. Addressing the problem of physician burnout is the shared responsibility of individual physicians and the organizations in which they work.

Adverse Events in Surgery

Over 51 million surgical procedures and operations were performed in the US in 2010 and the numbers are increasing each year [1]. Because of the critical and dynamic nature of many operative interventions, surgery accounts for a large number of the medical errors that occur every year. Despite improved therapies and technology, preventable medical errors and adverse events in surgery continue to occur and much interest is invested in this area to guide quality improvement efforts. Because reimbursements are being tied to quality outcomes in hospitals, these errors affect the income of the hospital and providers.

Research into iatrogenic injury over the last 3 decades has shed light on the rates of adverse events, characteristics, failure modes, and their sequelae. The California Medical

Association conducted the first large-scale study of adverse events in the 1970s when they reviewed the histories of 21,000 admissions and reported found that adverse events occurred in 4.6% [2]. The first study of surgical adverse events was performed by Couch et al. in 1981 who found that avoidable surgical errors occurred in more than 0.6% of their admissions to their academic general surgery service; 55% of these complications resulted in death [3]. In 1991, the Harvard Medical Practice Study published their retrospective analysis of 30,000 randomly selected patients and found an adverse event rate of 3.7%, many of which were a result of substandard care [4]. Since then, multiple studies have attempted to characterize these adverse events in an attempt to reduce the incidence of error. Gawande et al. analyzed the incidence and nature of adverse events in 15,000 patients in Colorado and Utah, finding that 66% of all adverse events were surgical, 54% were preventable, and 5.6% resulted in death. Technique-related complications, wound infections, and postoperative bleeding produced nearly half of all surgical adverse events [5]. Shortly after, a review of records from a population-based study in New York revealed that nearly 4% of hospitalized patients suffered adverse events. Two thirds of those events were considered to be caused by errors in management, most of which were not because of negligence [6].

Types of Surgical Errors

Patient safety problems of many kinds occur during the course of providing health care. They include transfusion errors, adverse drug events, wrong-site surgery, surgical injuries, hospital-acquired or other treatment-related infections, falls, burns, and pressure ulcers. Leap et al. characterized the kinds of errors that resulted in medical injury in the Medical Practice Study into groups including diagnostic, treatment, preventative, or other errors (Fig. 9.1) [6].

In any given patient, some or all of the types of errors can occur in a single hospitalization. A significant reason why adverse events occur in today's advanced medical system is

Diagnostic
  Error or delay in diagnosis
  Failure to employ indicated tests
  Use of outmoded tests or therapy
  Failure to act on results of monitoring or testing

Treatment
  Error in the performance of an operation, procedure, or test
  Error in administering the treatment
  Error in the dose or method of using a drug
  Avoidable delay in treatment or in responding to an abnormal test
  Inappropriate (not indicated) care

Preventative
  Failure to provide prophylactic treatment
  Inadequate monitoring or follow-up of treatment

Other
  Failure of communication
  Equipment failure
  Other system failure

FIG. 9.1 Types of surgical errors

that medical care is extremely complex and variable, involving a variety of personnel, equipment, and procedures [6]. Systems-based programs and solutions have been created and implemented and continuing efforts are in place to improve these approaches. These errors are being followed and reported by Hospital Systems. This chapter discusses the current topics around patient safety including government initiatives, public reporting, human factors in surgery, and surgery checklists, crew resource management, and resident duty hours, and physician burnout.

Initiatives around Patient Safety and Quality

More than a decade ago, the Institute of Medicine Quality of Healthcare in America Committee was formed to develop a strategy to improve quality. They released a comprehensive report "To Err is Human: Building a Safer Health System," addressing issues related to patient safety and laying out an ambitious national agenda for reducing errors in health care and improving patient safety [7]. Subsequently in 2005, the Patient Safety and Quality Improvement Act was signed into law to promote voluntary and confidential reporting of adverse events and improved communication between providers to improve patient safety [8]. Not long before that, the Medicare Prescription Drug, Improvement, and Modernization Act introduced the Acute Care Episode Demonstration, which aimed to shift the health care focus from quantity of care to quality of care [9]. The initiative resulted in millions of dollars saved without negatively impacting the patient safety [10, 11]. The most significant regulatory overhaul, however, was in 2010 when the Patient Protection and Affordable Care Act (PPACA) was signed into place. Under this act, the Center for Medicare and Medicaid (CMS) Innovation was established to improve quality of care and reduce the rate of growth in healthcare costs [12]. This resulted in further expansions of bundled payments and reimbursement shifts laid out by the CMS with the Innovation's Bundled Payments for Care Improvement Initiative (BPCI) as the most recent nation-wide project [13].

Linking Quality to Payment

The BPCI initiative links payments for multiple services received during a single episode of care with financial incentives for improved performance. The anticipation is that this model will lead to higher health care quality and more coordinated care at a lower cost. Traditionally, payments were made based on the fee-for-service (FFS) model, where institutions and providers were reimbursed for each individual service furnished to beneficiaries for a course of treatment. This resulted in fragmented care with minimal coordination between multidisciplinary providers, which led to a decrease in health care value; higher cost without improvement in patient outcomes. In 2013, the CMS announced their new shift in reimbursement mechanisms from the traditional FFS to the current proposed BPCI model with payment shifts based on the BPCI model to 30% by 2016 and to 50% by 2018, with the remaining FFS payments linked to institutions quality data to 90% by 2018 [13].

What is meant by quality data? Currently, three main programs exist to reward hospitals for delivering services of higher quality while penalizing those who do not meet performance benchmarks: The Hospital Readmissions Program, Hospital Value-Based Purchasing (HVBP) program, and Hospital Acquired Conditions (HAC). Since 2012, the Hospital Readmissions Reduction Program reduces payments to acute care hospitals with excess readmissions that are paid under the CMS's Inpatient Prospective Payment System. The excess readmission ratio is defined as the risk-adjusted predicted readmissions divided by the risk-adjusted expected readmissions. The payment adjustment amount is determined based on specific formulas based on DRGs and indirect costs [14]. The HVBP, also established by the Affordable Care Act, implements a pay-for-performance (P4P) approach to the payment system that accounts for the largest share of Medicare spending. Under the HVBP, Medicare adjusts a portion of payments to hospitals based on how well they perform on specific measures compared to other hospitals and how much they improve their own performance on those measures compared to their performance during a prior baseline period. The HVBP score is derived from The Total Performance Score (TPS), which consists of four domains—Clinical Process of Care, Patient Experience of Care, Outcome, and Efficiency domains (Table 9.1) [15]. The HVBP is designed to promote better clinical outcomes for hospitalized patients and improve their experience of care during hospital stays. Note that patient satisfaction is part of this composite and is becoming an ever larger part of the P4P picture and should be taken into account by the practitioner and the hospital.

The HAC Program reduces payments to hospitals that rank in the worst performing quartile. The worst performing quartile is identified by calculating the Total HAC score which is based on the hospital's performance on four risk-

TABLE 9.1 Domains of TPS for VBP

Domains of TPS for VBP	Composites	% of TPS
Clinical process of care domain	12 clinical process measures	10
Patient experience of care domain	8 dimensions of HCAHPS Survey	25
Outcome domain	3 mortality, 1 AHRQ, 1 HAI measure	40
Efficiency domain	1 Medicare Spending per Beneficiary	25

HCAHPS Hospital Consumer Assessment of Healthcare Providers and Systems, *HAI* Healthcare Associated Infection

adjusted quality measures (Patient Safety Indicator 90 composite, central-line-associated bloodstream infection (CLABSI), catheter-associated urinary tract infection (CAUTI), and surgical site infection (SSI) for colon surgery and hysterectomy). Hospitals with a total HAC score above 75th percentile of the Total HAC Score distribution may be subject to payment reduction [16].

Quality Improvement Programs

Several surgical quality improvement programs have been formed as a result of the increasing pressures and demands for improved patient safety and outcome in the health care environment. The Agency for Healthcare Research and Quality (AHRQ) developed four modules of Quality Indicators (QIs) to gauge performance in health care: the Prevention Quality Indicators (PQIs) [17], the Inpatient Quality Indicators (IQIs) [18], the Patient Safety Indicators (PSIs) [19], and the Pediatric Quality Indicators (PDIs)™. This chapter will focus on PSIs, which are quality measures that use administrative data based on the ICD-9-CM coding system found in discharge records. PSIs were developed to help hospitals identify potential adverse events to provide opportunity to assess incidences of adverse events and hospital complications [20]. There are currently 27 PSIs: 20 on the provider-level and 7 on the area-level. At the provider-level, the PSIs provide information about the potentially preventable complication patients experienced during their initial hospitalization (Table 9.2). The area-level PSIs capture all cases of potentially preventable complications that occur in a given geographical area (e.g. metropolitan service area or

TABLE 9.2 Patient Safety Indicators

Patient safety indicator: provider—level	PSI Number
Complications of anesthesia	1
Death in low-mortality DRGs	2
Decubitus ulcer	3
Failure to rescue	4
Foreign body left during procedure	5
Iatrogenic pneumothorax	6
Selected infections due to medical care	7
Postoperative hip fracture	8
Postoperative hemorrhage or hematoma	9
Postoperative physiologic and metabolic derangements	10
Postoperative respiratory failure	11
Postoperative pulmonary embolism or deep vein thrombosis	12
Postoperative sepsis	13
Postoperative wound dehiscence	14
Accidental puncture or laceration	15
Transfusion reaction	16
Birth trauma—injury to neonate	17
Obstetric trauma—vaginal with instrument	18
Obstetric trauma—vaginal without instrument	19
Obstetric trauma—cesarean delivery	20
Foreign body left during procedure	21
Iatrogenic pneumothorax	22
Selected infections due to medical care	23
Postoperative wound dehiscence	24
Accidental puncture or laceration	25
Transfusion reaction	26
Postoperative hemorrhage or hematoma	27

county) either during hospitalization or resulting in subsequent hospitalizations [19].

The AHRQ PSIs were initially designed as an internal quality improvement tool, but their use now ranges from public reporting to P4P initiatives. These indicators must be used with care as these are associated with limitations including coding inconsistencies, clinical vagueness in description of code, heterogeneity of clinical conditions, and incomplete or inaccurate administrative data. Many research efforts have been undertaken to validate the effectiveness in PSI's ability to capture potentially preventable patient safety events. While many PSIs have been shown to be unreliable as a detector of adverse events and a measure of quality performance, they are currently being used to present a picture of patient safety within all hospitals [21–25].

The American College of Surgeons National Surgical Quality Improvement Program (ACS NSQIP) is a nationally validated, risk-adjusted database tracking surgical outcomes. The program reports on a number of general surgical complications across multiple specialties and procedure-specific outcomes for a variety of individual procedures. The program allows participating institutions to view their benchmarked risk-adjusted parameters in order to develop goals and targets to decrease complications and mortalities. Similarly, the University HealthSystem Consortium (UHC) is another database available to subscribers, which provides benchmarked data comparative to other academic medical centers on safety, quality, and performance. Other available discipline-specific national outcomes databases include the Society for Thoracic Surgeons (STS) National Database, Tracking Operations Outcomes for Plastic Surgeons (TOPS) [26], and National Cancer Database (NCDB) [27] to name a few. All these tools will continue to be developed with the goal of providing sources for institutional improvements in patient safety while increasing transparency [27, 28].

Despite the advances in quality reporting, participation in nationally validated databases alone does not improve surgical outcomes. This was shown in a study conducted by Osborne et al. where they set out to evaluate the association

of enrollment in participation in the ACS NSQIP with outcomes. They found that after accounting for patient factors
and time trends toward improved outcomes, there was no
statistically significant improvement in outcomes at 1, 2, or
3 years after enrollment in ACS NSQIP [28]. They concluded
that feedback of outcomes data alone is not sufficient for
improving surgical outcomes. Failure to implement quality
improvement initiatives following review of ACS NSQIP
report may play a role in lack of progress. Because the ACS
NSQIP data is not publicly reported, institutions may not
have a large enough incentive to drive quality improvement.
Financial incentives are currently being implemented with
the BPCI initiative, pay-for-performance, and nonpayment
for adverse events. While change begins with the individual,
physicians may not have resources to launch effective programs.
Changing physician practice to adhere to quality improvement initiatives requires complex, multifaceted interventions
that need to be championed and sustained by the system. To
develop systematic approaches, the understanding of the
interplay between human factors and adverse events in a
system is crucial.

Human Factors in Surgery

Human error is inevitable in any discipline. While human error
oftentimes go unnoticed and rarely cause significant harm, the
occasions where they do translate into an adverse event cause
much distress in the system. It is known that although the individual commits human errors, the system is usually at fault for
inadequate organizational structures in not noticing the error
occurred. Much work has been done in the arena of human
factors of error, especially in the medical and surgical communities to detect vulnerable systems with the aim of reducing
error and optimizing patient safety. Three principles exist to
aid systems in their approach to understanding surgical errors;
(1) human error is unavoidable, (2) defective systems allow
human error to cause harm to the patient, and (3) systems can

be designed to prevent or detect human error before the patient is harmed [29].

One of the most well-known human factors theories is the "Swiss cheese" model of accident causation, which provides a framework for how errors or accidents occur in a system designed to deflect error. In this theory, systematic defenses exist to prevent error; however, occasionally each specific event (e.g. organizational factors, unsafe supervision, preconditions for unsafe acts, or the unsafe act itself) at a given time and place lines up such that the event bypasses the system's defenses and translates into an error (Fig. 9.2) [30]. Therefore, preventable adverse events, despite committed by individuals, are rather a result of a defective system.

The Systems Engineering Initiative for Patient Safety Model (SEIP) effectively describes a system that is relevant to the surgical process (Fig. 9.3) [31]. The framework aids in understanding the structures, processes, and outcomes in a health care system. The model places the patient in the center while all the elements of the system not only affect the patient, but also affects the other elements within the system. The model implies that overall quality, patient safety, and outcomes are affected by the interplay between factors such as teamwork and communication, physical work environment, technology, workload factors, and other organizational variables. Specifically, in the operating room, environmental factors such as clutter, noise, lighting, and temperature can negatively impact the outcome of an operation [32–34]. Poor communication has also been shown to be the cause of a large number of sentinel events within the healthcare system with studies revealing that 40% of errors in surgery resulted from communication errors [35, 36]. From a technology standpoint, the advancements in minimally invasive and robotic surgery require new skill sets to be learned which, when combined with the other systematic elements, may be a source for stress-inducing conditions. Thus, operating rooms designed to effectively link these elements to prevent or detect human error before a patient is harmed will succeed in providing coordinated, effective, efficient, and safe surgery.

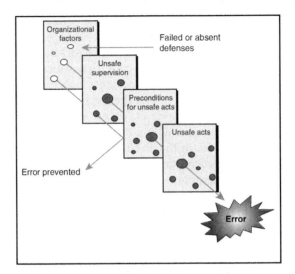

Fɪɢ. 9.2 Swiss cheese model of accident error causation

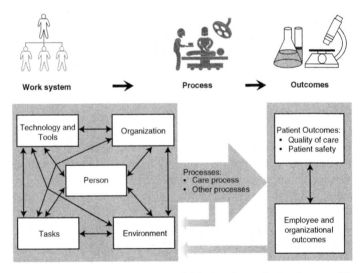

Fɪɢ. 9.3 The systems engineering initiative for patient safety model

Crew Resource Management

Communication plays a significant role in a success of a team, especially in the operating room. The well-known strategy, Crew Resource Management (CRM), developed in the aviation industry has been successfully adapted in some hospital systems to improve quality and safety. At one institution, The Ohio State University Wexner Medical Center, CRM was translated to the healthcare industry as a systematic approach to training leadership, staff, and physicians on the elements of communication, conflict management, safety tools, and internal monitoring. Safety tools include checklists, standardized protocols, and communication scripts. Within 3 years following CRM implementation, the health system reduced their total number of adverse events by 27.5% [37]. In another study, Funai et al. incrementally introduced multiple patient safety interventions at a university-based obstetrics service. The initiative included outside expert review, protocol standardization, creation of a patient safety nurse position and patient safety committee, and training in team skills and fetal heart monitoring interpretation. They reported significantly reduced adverse outcomes following intervention with significant improvement in the safety climate [38]. This demonstrates the measurable outcomes, effectiveness, and feasibility of a communication-based training program in improving patient safety.

Surgical Checklists

The implementation of checklists and standardized processes around the care of patients has been pivotal to the development of the patient safety culture [39]. Dr. Pronovost and his team at John's Hopkins were the first to pioneer a rounding checklist in the Intensive Care Unit (ICU) aimed at decreasing catheter-related bloodstream infections. In his cohort study of 103 ICU's, 1981 ICU days, and 373,757 catheter-days, he found that the use of the ICU checklist resulted in a sustained reduction of 66% in rates of catheter-related bloodstream infections [40].

In 2009, the World Health Organization issued a worldwide recommendation for the use of its surgical safety checklist for briefings in the operating room, which included a "sign in" immediately before induction of anesthesia, a "time out" immediately before the skin incision, and a "sign-out" following skin closure. The WHO checklist was evaluated in a study of eight hospitals in different parts of the world and was shown to result in a significant reduction of mortality in major surgery by 47% and a significant relative reduction of major morbidity by 36% [39]. Results from a meta-analysis including 20 studies concerning the effect of the WHO checklist on safety-related events in the OR support the WHO's recommendation to use the Surgical Safety Checklist in all operative procedures [41]. Institutions can create individual adaptations of content, form, and model of the checklist as long as the purpose remains the structured communication among team members regarding important information related to the procedure. Since then, checklists have been implemented during bedside procedures, obstetric processes, trauma cases in the Emergency Department, as well as patient handoffs between residents and nurses. Ultimately, the use of checklists and its success is entirely dependent on the implementation and monitoring from the institution as well as the collaboration of all health care providers.

Duty Hours and Physician Burnout

The introduction of the mandated work hour restrictions, introduced in July 2003 by the Accreditation Council for Graduate Medical Education (ACGME), was designed to improve patient safety by reducing resident fatigue. Since then, much interest has been placed in evaluating the effects of duty hour restrictions on patient safety. A 2012 survey indicated that most categorical surgery residents did not perceive that reduced duty hours noticeably improved quality of care, and their perceptions of causes of medical errors suggested that system changes were more likely to enhance patient safety than further hour limits [46]. Most recently, a national cluster-randomized trial comparing standard ACGME duty hours to more flexible policies (waived rules on maximum shift lengths and time off between shifts) was completed to assess differences in patient outcomes, resident education, and well-being. Results including 117 general surgery programs in the US between 2014 and 2015 demonstrated no significant difference in residents' satisfaction with overall well-being and education quality between the two duty hour policies [47]. These results question whether current ACGME duty hour restrictions provide residents with the optimal surgical training while balancing resident well-being with patient safety and outcomes.

In addition to balancing work hours, Hospital Systems are now faced with alarming rates of burnout among physician providers. National studies suggest that at least 50% of US physicians are experiencing professional burnout [48–50]. Burnout is characterized by exhaustion, depersonalization, cynicism, low sense of personal accomplishment, and reduced effectiveness. Physician burnout has been shown to impair job performance and influence quality of care, patient safety, and patient satisfaction [51–53]. Consequently, there has been a rising interest in interventional strategies focused on improving physician wellness. Individual stress reduction strategies have proved to be effective in healthcare professionals [54, 55]. However, mitigating professional burnout is not solely the responsibility of the individual physician but that of the entire hospital organization. In addition to providing resources to promote self-care and resilience, much work remains in developing sustained systematic strategies to harness physician wellness that will in turn impact safety and quality for patients.

Conclusions

The goal of any institution healthcare institution is to eliminate errors and improve patient safety. Over the last decade, much effort has been placed in this endeavor with significant success as indicated by results from CRM training and checklist implementation. Governmental quality improvement initiatives and systematic strategies have been developed to provide safe, timely, efficient, effective, equitable, and patient-centered care. These proposals now hold health care institutions and providers accountable for achieving the quadruple aim in healthcare: to enhance the patient's experience by improving costs, quality, and outcomes, while maintaining physician well-being. With increasing awareness and accountability, compliance has become less of an issue. What remains now is sustainability and growth of a culture around patient-safety.

References

1. Centers for Disease Control and Prevention. National Hospital Discharge Survey: 2010 table, Procedures by selected patient characteristics — number by procedure category and age. Atlanta: CDC; 2010.
2. Mills DH. Report of the medical insurance feasibility study. San Francisco: California Medical Association; 1977.
3. Couch NP, Tilney NL, Rayner AA, Moore FD. The high cost of low-frequency events: the anatomy and economics of surgical mishaps. N Engl J Med. 1981;304(11):634–7.
4. Brennan TA, Leape LL, Laird NM, et al. Incidence of adverse events and negligence in hospitalized patients: results of the Harvard Medical Practice Study I. 1991. Qual Saf Health Care. 2004;13(2):145–51. discussion 151–42
5. Gawande AA, Thomas EJ, Zinner MJ, Brennan TA. The incidence and nature of surgical adverse events in Colorado and Utah in 1992. Surgery. 1999;126(1):66–75.
6. Leape LL, Lawthers AG, Brennan TA, Johnson WG. Preventing medical injury. QRB Qual Rev Bull. 1993;19(5):144–9.

7. Kohn LT, Corrigan JM, Donaldson MS, editors. To err is human: building a safer health system. Washington: National Academies Press; 2000.

8. AHRQ. Patient Safety and Quality Improvement Act of 2005. Agency for Healthcare Research and Quality; 2008. http://archive.ahrq.gov/news/newsroom/press-releases/2008/psoact.html.

9. Center for Medicare and Medicaid. Acute care episode demonstration. http://archive.ahrq.gov/news/newsroom/press-releases/2008/psoact.html. 2008.

10. Herman B. 2 major lessons from CMS' bundled payment ACE demonstration. Becker's Hospital Review. http://www.beckershospitalreview.com/hospital-physician-relationships/2-major-lessons-from-CMS-bundled-payment-ace-demonstration.html.

11. Vesely R. An ACE in the deck? Bundled-payment demo shows returns. Mod Healthc. 2011;41(6):32–3.

12. U.S. Department of Health & Human Services. Key features of the affordable care act by year. http://www.hhs.gov/healthcare/facts-and-features/key-features-of-aca-by-year/index.html. Accessed Nov 22, 2015.

13. Bundled Payments for Care Iniative (BCPI) overview: general information. Center for Medicare and Medicaid Services. http://innovation.cms.gov/initiatives/bundled-payments/.

14. Centers for Medicare and Medicaid Services. Readmissions reduction program. https://www.cms.gov/Medicare/Medicare-Fee-for-Service-Payment/AcuteInpatientPPS/Readmissions-Reduction-Program.html. Accessed Nov 22, 2015.

15. The Official U.S. Government Site for Medicare. https://www.medicare.gov/hospitalcompare/data/total-performance-scores.html. 2015.

16. Hospital-acquired Condition Reduction Program. The Official U.S. Government Site for Medicare. https://www.medicare.gov/hospitalcompare/HAC-reduction-program.html. Accessed Nov 22, 2015.

17. AHRQ. Guide to the prevention quality indicators. Agency for Healthcare Research and Quality 2006; Sages Patient Safety Chapter 11.22.docx Accessed Nov 22, 2015.

18. AHRQ. Guide to inpatient quality indicators. Agency for Healthcare Research and Quality 2006. http://www.qualityindicators.ahrq.gov/Downloads/Modules/IQI/V30/iqi_guide_v30.pdf. Accessed Nov 22, 2015.

19. AHRQ. Guide to patient safety indicators. AHRQ for Healthcare Research and Quality 2007; http://www.qualityindicators.ahrq.gov/Downloads/Modules/PSI/V31/psi_guide_v31.pdf. Accessed Nov 22, 2015.

20. AHRQ. Agency for Healthcare Research and Quality. U.S. Department of Health & Human Services. http://www.ahrq.gov, 2015.

21. Cima RR, Lackore KA, Nehring SA, et al. How best to measure surgical quality? Comparison of the Agency for Healthcare Research and Quality Patient Safety Indicators (AHRQ-PSI) and the American College of Surgeons National Surgical Quality Improvement Program (ACS-NSQIP) postoperative adverse events at a single institution. Surgery. 2011;150(5):943–9.

22. Kaafarani HM, Borzecki AM, Itani KM, et al. Validity of selected Patient Safety Indicators: opportunities and concerns. J Am Coll Surg. 2011;212(6):924–34.

23. Koch CG, Li L, Hixson E, Tang A, Phillips S, Henderson JM. What are the real rates of postoperative complications: elucidating inconsistencies between administrative and clinical data sources. J Am Coll Surg. 2012;214(5):798–805.

24. Romano PS, Mull HJ, Rivard PE, et al. Validity of selected AHRQ patient safety indicators based on VA National Surgical Quality Improvement Program data. Health Serv Res. 2009;44(1):182–204.

25. Utter GH, Cuny J, Strater A, Silver MR, Hossli S, Romano PS. Variation in academic medical centers' coding practices for postoperative respiratory complications: implications for the AHRQ postoperative respiratory failure Patient Safety Indicator. Med Care. 2012;50(9):792–800.

26. TOPS (Tracking Operations and Outcomes for Plastic Surgeons). American Society of Plastic Surgeons. http://www.plasticsurgery.org/for-medical-professionals/quality-and-health-policy/tops.html. Accessed Nov 22, 2015.

27. American College of Surgeons. National Cancer Data Base. https://www.facs.org/quality programs/cancer/ncdb. Accessed Nov 22, 2015.

28. Osborne NH, Nicholas LH, Ryan AM, Thumma JR, Dimick JB. Association of hospital participation in a quality reporting program with surgical outcomes and expenditures for Medicare beneficiaries. JAMA. 2015;313(5):496–504.

29. Etchells E, O'Neill C, Bernstein M. Patient safety in surgery: error detection and prevention. World J Surg. 2003;27(8):936–41. discussion 941–32

30. Weigmann D, Shappell S. A human error approach to aviation accident analysis: the human factors analysis and classification system. Farnham: Ashgate; 2003.
31. Carayon P, Schoofs Hundt A, Karsh BT, et al. Work system design for patient safety: the SEIPS model. Qual Saf Health Care. 2006;15(Suppl 1):i50–8.
32. Fanning J. Illumination in the operating room. Biomed Instrum Technol. 2005;39(5):361–2.
33. Healey AN, Sevdalis N, Vincent CA. Measuring intra-operative interference from distraction and interruption observed in the operating theatre. Ergonomics. 2006;49(5–6):589–604.
34. Ofek E, Pizov R, Bitterman N. From a radial operating theatre to a self-contained operating table. Anaesthesia. 2006;61(6):548–52.
35. Lingard L, Regehr G, Orser B, et al. Evaluation of a preoperative checklist and team briefing among surgeons, nurses, and anesthesiologists to reduce failures in communication. Arch Surg. 2008;143(1):12–7. discussion 18
36. Gawande AA, Zinner MJ, Studdert DM, Brennan TA. Analysis of errors reported by surgeons at three teaching hospitals. Surgery. 2003;133(6):614–21.
37. Moffatt-Bruce SD, Hefner JL, Mekhjian H, et al. What is the return on investment for implementation of a crew resource management program at an Academic Medical Center? Am J Med Qual. 2015.
38. Pettker CM, Thung SF, Norwitz ER, et al. Impact of a comprehensive patient safety strategy on obstetric adverse events. Am J Obstet Gynecol. 2009;200(5):492.e1–8.
39. Haynes AB, Weiser TG, Berry WR, et al. A surgical safety checklist to reduce morbidity and mortality in a global population. N Engl J Med. 2009;360(5):491–9.
40. Pronovost P, Needham D, Berenholtz S, et al. An intervention to decrease catheter-related bloodstream infections in the ICU. N Engl J Med. 2006;355(26):2725–32.
41. Fudickar A, Horle K, Wiltfang J, Bein B. The effect of the WHO Surgical Safety Checklist on complication rate and communication. Dtsch Arztebl Int. 2012;109(42):695–701.
42. Gelfand DV, Podnos YD, Carmichael JC, Saltzman DJ, Wilson SE, Williams RA. Effect of the 80-hour workweek on resident burnout. Arch Surg. 2004;139(9):933–8. discussion 938–40
43. Wetzel CM, Kneebone RL, Woloshynowych M, et al. The effects of stress on surgical performance. Am J Surg. 2006;191(1):5–10.

44. Wiggins-Dohlvik K, Stewart RM, Babbitt RJ, Gelfond J, Zarzabal LA, Willis RE. Surgeons' performance during critical situations: competence, confidence, and composure. Am J Surg. 2009; 198(6):817–23.

45. Wetzel CM, Black SA, Hanna GB, et al. The effects of stress and coping on surgical performance during simulations. Ann Surg. 2010;251(1):171–6.

46. Borman KR, Jones AT, Shea JA. Duty hours, quality of care, and patient safety: general surgery resident perceptions. J Am Coll Surg. 2012;215(1):70–7. discussion 77–9

47. Bilimoria KY, Chung JW, Hedges LV, et al. National cluster-randomized trial of duty-hour flexibility in surgical training. N Engl J Med. 2016;374(8):713–27.

48. Maslach C, Jackson SE. Burnout in health professionals: a social psychological analysis. Social Psychology of Health and Illness: Hillsdale; 1982.

49. Elmore LC, Jeffe DB, Jin L, Awad MM, Turnbull IR. National Survey of Burnout among US General Surgery Residents. J Am Coll Surg. 2016;223(3):440–51.

50. Medscape 2016: Bias and burnout. Lifestyle Report. http://www.medscape.com/features/slideshow/lifestyle/2016/public/overview. Accessed Sept 30, 2016.

51. Gundersen L. Physician burnout. Ann Intern Med. 2001; 135(2):145–8.

52. O'Connor PG, Spickard Jr A. Physician impairment by substance abuse. Med Clin North Am. 1997;81(4):1037–52.

53. Vaillant GE, Sobowale NC, McArthur C. Some psychologic vulnerabilities of physicians. N Engl J Med. 1972;287(8):372–5.

54. Olson K, Kemper KJ, Mahan JD. What factors promote resilience and protect against burnout in first-year pediatric and medicine-pediatric residents? J Evid Based Complementary Altern Med. 2015;20(3):192–8.

55. Kemper KJ, Khirallah M. Acute effects of online mind-body skills training on resilience, mindfulness, and empathy. J Evid Based Complementary Altern Med. 2015;20(4):247–53.

Chapter 10
Strategies to Help Establish Your Practice While Simultaneously Achieving Work Life Balance

Denise W. Gee and Yulia Zak

Work hour restrictions do not exist beyond formal training programs. In addition, while many hospital-based practices continue to explore various clinical coverage arrangements for weekends and holidays, most practicing surgeons carry the sole responsibility of care for their own patients for the duration of their career. The reality of a surgeon's life is that we work harder and often with longer hours than is currently allowed in residency training. Nevertheless, we have access to some crucial tools that can make such a busy life significantly more manageable and very fulfilling.

There exists no foolproof recipe or algorithm for success. Perhaps more importantly, every surgeon's definition of success is unique and will likely change over time. In this chapter, we discuss key strategies that can facilitate a smooth transition

D.W. Gee, M.D. (✉)
Massachusetts General Hospital, Division of General and Gastrointestinal Surgery, Boston, MA, USA
e-mail: dgee@mgh.harvard.edu

Y. Zak, M.D.
Department of Surgery, Icahn School of Medicine at Mount Sinai, New York, NY, USA

© Springer International Publishing AG 2017
D.B. Renton et al. (eds.), *The SAGES Manual Transitioning to Practice*, DOI 10.1007/978-3-319-51397-3_10

145

from the training environment to a clinically busy but well-balanced practice and life in the field of surgery.

Optimizing the Transition to Practice

One of the first things to do after you graduate from residency or fellowship is to make sure you have identified a potential mentor(s) among your established colleagues. This person should be willing to guide you through the process of establishing your practice, whether it is networking with referring providers in private practice or navigating the academic ladder in a university setting. No matter how well-trained you are, there will be times when you will need a skilled assistant during a tougher-than-expected case or someone to run your difficult cases by. In addition to developing a mentorship in your new workplace, take full advantage of the relationships you have already established in residency and fellowship. Your former teachers can and will be incredible resources in your clinical decision-making process, as well as in serving as references for society memberships, committees, and future jobs.

As you start your practice, carefully consider your desired case mix and what subspecialty reputation you plan to establish for yourself. It will be easier to grow your practice initially if you encourage referrals of patients with a wide range of pathology that falls within the scope of your general surgery training. This is especially true for surgeons in the community setting. On the other hand, if your goal is to establish yourself as a subspecialist with fellowship training, you are more likely to set yourself apart from the other general surgeons in the area and receive more complex referrals within your field of expertise. Developing a niche will allow you to hone your skills in a particular area, facilitate research on related topics, and build your reputation as a leader in that field [2]. From a practical standpoint, remember to bring your residency/fellowship program's post-operative order sets, perioperative treatment protocols, and operating room preference cards/lists to ensure that your patients will get cared for in the manner in which you have become accustomed to. This will facilitate efficient transition into practice without wasting time to reinvent the wheel [1].

In addition to carefully choosing clinical mentors and associates, surgeons in community practice will especially benefit from the selection of qualified business advisors, attorneys, and accountants who can potentially ease the transition process. Most surgeons at the end of their training do not have a sufficient business background to immediately create a thriving practice. Surrounding yourself with trustworthy and experienced businesspeople will provide invaluable learning opportunities and help you avoid potentially costly mistakes [3].

Cultivating Professional Connections

One of the most important tenets of a successful practice is to be affable and available. Unless you were lucky enough to inherit a thriving practice from a retiring surgeon, you will need to build a wide network of referring providers and establish yourself as a skilled surgeon with good outcomes and satisfied patients. Initially, this will require reaching out to the community physicians to let them know about your presence, credentials, and availability. Set aside some time to meet with individual providers in person. Offer the heads of adjoining departments to give Grand Rounds about topics within your field of expertise. Put together a CME course for the community PCPs and other referring providers. Visit outlying private practices or smaller hospitals and schedule lunch presentations for physicians and mid-level practitioners. Make sure to bring business cards, pamphlets, and any other marketing materials you can produce.

Once you begin receiving referrals, maintain ongoing communication with these providers, so they know what is happening with their patient. When you see a patient in clinic, always send a letter or email to the referring physician with your assessment and plan or call him/her directly with an update. Such letters can be based on templates to save you time. Some electronic medical records (EMRs) even have a streamlined pathway for faxing your progress notes with a few clicks of the mouse. Return all phone calls and emails promptly and never turn away a referral or a request for a transfer or help. Even if you are not able to help, facilitate advancing the patient's care to someone who can assist. The time invested in this will pay off with an increase in referrals (and revenue!) [4].

At the same time that you are busy building your practice, always remember that the colleagues in your practice/department are part of your team. You do not need to overextend yourself and risk burning out in an effort to try to take care of every patient and every problem. If there is a subspecialist who can do something better than you, refer appropriate patients to him/her. You will be viewed as a partner and a team-player and will receive referrals within your subspecialty in return. Most importantly, you will maintain your balance and sanity by minimizing your risk of complications and not trying to do every case in sight.

In the operating suites, always be polite and respectful to the staff. Often, a surgeon's behavior and actions are instrumental in setting the tone in the operating room. Never raise your voice or speak down to the nurses and never publicly criticize others. Building good relationships with the OR staff will pay off in the long run with a pleasant work environment. As you spend more time in the operating room, being a well-liked member of the team can positively impact your relationship with OR administration as well, potentially resulting in improved operative help, as well as assistance with placing add-on cases as efficiently as possible.

Leading a Team

If at all possible, participate in the hiring or selection process of your support staff. Prioritize choosing candidates with excellent communication skills and experience in similar positions. Set clear expectations from the very beginning and ensure that your treatment protocols are known and followed. Review workflow pathways and look for opportunities to streamline flow of information to minimize omissions and delays. Your support staff's attention to detail will influence your ability to be efficient. For example, make sure that all incoming lab and test results are checked regularly and delivered to your inbox, and surgical pathology results are included in the patient's chart at the time of postoperative follow-up. Your staff should know that you have a policy of never turning patients away, and that the highest quality of care is your primary goal. At the same time, give them ample notice to modify your clinic schedule if you have prior family or social commitments, let them know when you need to cut clinic short in order to make your child's soccer game, and allow them to be creative in scheduling in order to accommodate patients in a timely fashion. This may mean having special office hours if you have missed a clinic.

Unlike the work hours of your staff, expectations of you and your time can be unlimited. In order to balance clinical practice, potential administrative or educational duties, research, and family commitments, one must develop a schedule that integrates all of these components [4]. Ensure that both your administrative assistant (AA) and your significant other have access to your calendar (without sharing HIPAA-protected or other sensitive information). Be sure to block off time for billing, answering emails, performing research, and attending to family obligations just as you would for OR cases or other work meetings. Your AA should be invested in protecting your personal time as much as they are in maximizing patient satisfaction and your efficiency. On the other hand, maintaining a centralized schedule will also allow your staff to more easily reach you for emergencies.

You will need to set the trend for the atmosphere and mood that prevails in your practice. A grumpy surgeon soon begets unhappy staff, and this trickles down to the patients and referring physicians. However, it is not enough for you alone to be affable. Your team represents you and often interacts with the patients even more than you do in an outpatient setting. Set the precedent for courteous, amiable communication with your staff, and let them know that it is a priority to maintain the same type of rapport with patients, families, and other physicians. Show your team that you value their work, and make sure they have enough time off to stay fresh, interested, and amiable.

Once you have an established busy practice, this may be the time to consider hiring a mid-level provider. A physician assistant or nurse practitioner can be instrumental in increasing the efficiency of your clinic evaluations. She/he can also take a significant portion of the paperwork burden off your shoulders and streamline communication with patients. This may allow you to increase your productivity while actually cutting back on your work hours, reducing the risk of burnout, and improving your job satisfaction by allowing you to focus on what you love to do best—operate and take care of sick patients. A scribe may also be beneficial in your practice, allowing you to spend more time talking to the patient in clinic and less time worrying about chart documentation.

Finally, be proud of your accomplishments and make sure your superiors are aware of the hard work that you do. When it is time to re-negotiate your contract, do not hesitate to ask for any additional resources that may improve your clinical and academic output and help to better balance your life. In the end, being a team player is critical and if you are fulfilling all of your obligations, it is important for your department to support you in a similar fashion.

Staying Current and Skilled

In order to maximize the longevity of your career and the quality of the care you provide to your the patients, you must keep up with the current literature, research, and new technologies. Residency/fellowship should not be the end of your education. It is important to attend the American College of Surgeons and/or your subspecialty annual regional and national society meetings. Try to take at least one hands-on course per year to renew/refresh your skills or to learn a new technique altogether. Read surgical journals on a regular basis. Be curious about colleagues trying out new techniques or simply learn from them and perhaps adopt some of their "tricks". Regardless of how available or affable you are, nothing can or will substitute for your "ability", i.e. skills and knowledge set. Furthermore, just as your practice model and professional goals will change throughout your career, your skills must evolve to adopt new concepts and techniques to provide the best possible care for your patients [5]. This is critical to maintaining relevance and longevity in your practice.

Preserving your Passion

Throughout your career, if you can protect the joy you felt the first time you held a scalpel, you will be much less likely to burn out. Identify what keeps your surgical passion alive and cultivate it, keeping in mind that this may change over the years.

In the hospital, become involved in departmental and/or hospital-wide committees. This will help develop your leadership skills and facilitate change in the issues you feel strongly about.

Do not miss opportunities to teach. Whether you are at an academic institution or in private practice, sharing your knowledge and experience with students, residents, junior partners, or community physicians can be extraordinarily fulfilling and will give you a sense of a built legacy that will remain long after you take your last call.

Remember that you cannot be everything to everyone. Preserving work-life balance is crucial and reaching that balance can occur in many different permutations depending on the individual. Staying true to what your personal needs are, in both work and life, and striving to maintain them will keep you happier in the long run.

Maintaining a Healthy Personal Life

In the business world, there exists a concept of a kaleidoscope strategy. In this abstraction, there are four chambers in the kaleidoscope vision of a successful life: happiness, achievement, significance, and legacy. Each of these holds together elements pertaining to one's individuality, family, work, and community. It is thought that those who structure their goals by creating "chips" distributed among the four categories in a balanced way are much more likely to achieve enduring success in life [6].

For most surgeons, the time available to be spent with family or friends does not increase after finishing training and entering practice. However, the flexibility in how to spend that bonding time improves significantly, and consequently, the quality of life can surge.

First, you must protect family time without compromising patient care. Invest in a high-quality nighttime and weekend answering service for your practice. Ensure that you will be contacted immediately for urgent issues, while protecting your sleep and your family from the interruptions of non-emergent phone calls. If possible, do the same with work-related meetings, and schedule them for early morning, between cases, or over lunch [7].

Second, maintain an ongoing conversation with your partner or spouse about your mutual career goals and expectations regarding the distribution of responsibilities at home. As your career evolves, the amount and kind of obligations you are able to take on will also change. Reciprocal flexibility with the division of labor will allow both spouses to achieve success at work and at home. Whenever possible (and affordable), outsource the household chores that do not contribute to your relationships but actually take time away from them. At the same time, consider the needs of your family, such as employment prospects for your spouse, educational opportunities for your children, and options for recreation and travel, when choosing practice locations or organizations [3]. It will be much easier to focus on building a successful career when your family members' needs are met. Be sure to protect time to spend with your partner or spouse. In a setting of increased work and life demands, it can become easy to forget the needs of your significant other. Just as you block time for work commitments, make sure to set aside time to be with the person who is very likely your biggest supporter.

Third, if you plan on having children, realize that there will never be a "perfect" time to take this step. The most important elements in your success as a parent are flexibility, discipline, organization, and endurance. Slaughter proposes that career development with a family and children is akin to irregular stair steps with scattered plateaus and dips. One may occasionally have to turn down promotions to remain in a job that best suits the family situation, work part-time for a period of time, or take a sabbatical in order to put "money in the family bank" [8]. With a career that will likely span decades, remember that there will be plenty of time to achieve your professional goals without missing out on important experiences during the crucial years of parenting.

On the other hand, keep in mind that it is often possible to structure your life during the intensive years of building a successful clinical practice in a way that allows for responsible (and joyful) parenting. For example, instead of spending late evenings in the office catching up on paperwork, choose to go home for dinner with your family or to see your child's play recital, and then finish your work after the children have gone to sleep. Avoid scheduling meetings during the hours your children are not asleep or at school. You can choose to start your clinic after you have taken your daughter to school, or get up earlier in the morning to catch up on email so that you can have breakfast with your son. Schedule call as far in advance as possible, and avoid taking it during important family events. Conversely, when you are not on call, deliberately schedule family bonding opportunities. You may even consider combining society meetings with family getaways for maximum efficiency.

Next, become involved in your community. Volunteer for your children's school functions or sports events. Attend town hall meetings and participate in the neighborhood association initiatives. Not only will this bring you closer to your family, but it will also support your identity outside of work, help you make new friends and connections, and widen your social network. Community involvement could potentially bring in additional clinical referrals as well!

Finally, do not forget to take some time for yourself. Plan time for regular exercise and maintain a healthy lifestyle. Without your health, burnout at work will quickly strip you of personal and professional happiness. Taking care of yourself and maintaining your health is the most critical piece of the work-life balance puzzle.

Work-life balance in the life of an ambitious and successful surgeon will always be a moving target. Sir William Osler's concept of availability, affability, and ability is the common thread that ties together all the components of a meaningful and rewarding life. It applies not only to the professional arena, but to your family and personal life as well. Most of all, adapting to change while prioritizing those people and aspects of your professional and personal life that provide you with the most happiness will ensure that when you look back at your accomplishments 30 or 40 years from now, you will have no regrets and a legacy of cherished memories.

References

1. Althausen PL. Building a successful trauma practice in a community setting. J Orthop Trauma. 2011;25(Suppl 3):S113-7.
2. Stannard JP. Building a successful trauma practice in academics. J Orthop Trauma. 2011;25(suppl 3):S111-2.
3. Brandt MT. Transitioning from residency to private practice. Oral Maxillofac Surg Clin North Am. 2008;20(1):1-9.
4. Liporace FA. My first year in academic practice: what I learned, what I wish I knew, what I would do differently. J Orthop Trauma. 2011;25(suppl 3):S118-20.
5. Watson JT. Things you never thought of that make a difference: personal goals, common sense, and good behavior in practice. J Orthop Trauma. 2011;25(Suppl 3):S121-3.
6. Nash, L., Stevenson, H., Success that lasts. Harv Bus Rev. 2004(February): 102-9.
7. Murtha Y. Perspectives of being spouse, parent, and surgeon. J Orthop Trauma. 2013;27(suppl 1):S12-3.
8. Slaughter, A., Why women still can't have it all. The Atlantic. 2012. July/August: 85-102.

Chapter 11
Social Media and Networking in Surgical Practice

Erin Bresnahan, Adam C. Nelson, and Brian P. Jacob

Introduction

Social media (SM) has become an important means of communication allowing people from across the world to exchange ideas based upon their common interests. The use of SM has risen dramatically in a relatively short period of time and has quickly affected the way surgeons acquire and consume information. By embracing the transparency afforded by the platforms and the ability to globally collaborate in real time using smart phones, by using closed Facebook™ groups, surgeons have discovered a new way to educate each other, and in return optimize the treatments and outcomes for their patients (Fig. 11.1).

E. Bresnahan, B.A.
Icahn School of Medicine at Mount Sinai, New York, NY, USA

A.C. Nelson, M.D.
Department of General Surgery, Mount Sinai Hospital,
New York, NY, USA

B.P. Jacob, M.D. (✉)
Department of Surgery, Mount Sinai Health System,
1010 Fifth Ave, New York, NY 10028, USA
e-mail: bpjacob@gmail.com

© Springer International Publishing AG 2017
D.B. Renton et al. (eds.), *The SAGES Manual Transitioning to Practice*, DOI 10.1007/978-3-319-51397-3_11

155

Social Networking Use Has Shot Up in Past Decade

% of all American adults and internet-using adults who use at least one social networking site

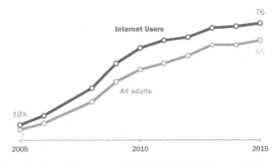

Source: Pew Research Center surveys. 2005-2006, 2008-2015. No data are available for 2007.

PEW RESEARCH CENTER

FIG. 11.1 The percentage of all American adults and Internet-using adults who use at least one social networking site

Usage of SM among medical professionals has been observed to mirror the growth trends of the general population. A 2010 nationwide survey reported SM use by 93.5% of medical students, 79.4% of residents, and 41.6% of practicing physicians [2]. While the majority of respondents used SM for personal purposes only, it is obvious that the exchange of information afforded by SM has numerous applications within the professional realm of surgery as well. Indeed, the role of SM in surgical practice is increasingly being advocated as a means of professional collaboration and as a way to augment the patient–doctor relationship [3]. With these new opportunities come challenging questions regarding ethics, patient privacy, and professionalism. Therefore, the goal of this chapter is to serve as guide to those who are transitioning into surgical practice by addressing the following:

- Definition and explanation of SM
- How can SM benefit surgeons?

- How can SM benefit patients?
- How does one maintain professionalism and compliance?
- Specific examples of SM as a tool in surgical practice

Definition of Social Media

Social media refers to websites where users can both post content and generate discussion, with the end goal being to engage audiences and facilitate relationships. The total number and variety of SM platforms can seem endless; however, a handful of platforms have consistently been among the most popular over several years (Fig. 11.2). Facebook continues to be the most used SM platform with 71% of Internet users having an account [4]. While the growth of Facebook has shown little change over the past few years,

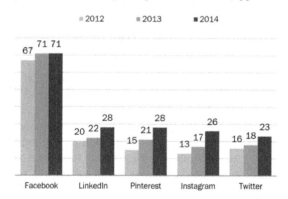

Social media sites, 2012-2014

% of online adults who use the following social media websites, by year

Pew Research Center's Internet Project Surveys, 2012-2014. 2014 data collected September 11-14 & September 18-21, 2014. N=1,597 internet users ages 18+.

PEW RESEARCH CENTER

FIG. 11.2 The percentage of online adults who use the following social media websites, by year

growth of other popular SM platforms (LinkedIn, Pinterest, Instagram, and Twitter) has been increasing steadily. Furthermore, the number of adults who use more than one SMN platform is rapidly increasing, up to 52% in 2014 [4]. Other platforms are also considered social media, like rating websites, blogs, and even Google, in the sense that all of these sites offer a platform where transparent dialogue can be posted in real time.

Also important to consider is the way in which people are accessing these platforms. Usage on mobile devices has increased considerably, meaning that more people can have access to social media at times when they are not tied down to a computer—which offers great potential for reaching busy physicians. The ability to scroll through a newsfeed while grabbing lunch in the cafeteria, or read an article someone posted while on the train, enables an audience of busy professionals to connect more frequently with others on SM during breaks in their schedule, through the freedom of mobile usage.

The ease of access of social media websites as well as the widespread network of daily users already in place makes social media an optimal platform for connecting physicians with patients, physicians with others in their field, patients with other patients, and patients with information about their health and illnesses. People are more likely to read something or accommodate it into their practice if it is easy to access and if the information is channeled through means that are already incorporated into their daily routines. A large percentage of the population checks their social media accounts daily, so information posted to these sites would reach many more people than that of a site which had to start from the bottom up in first recruiting users and then working up enough engagement to support daily usage.

In addition to the mainstream platforms mentioned above, there are a multitude of smaller, niche sites which target a more specific audience. Such platforms are increasingly being used for health-related purposes. For example, Chronology

[5] is a social media network (SMN) patient-to-patient network specifically for people with Crohn's disease, which features a "health timeline" where patients log their symptoms over time alongside the various treatments they have used. Not only can patients use these niche sites, but physicians are employing their use as well, to interact with or provide information and support to the communities they serve.

How Can SMN Benefit Surgeons?

SMN is now being used to establish an online presence for surgical practices and healthcare organizations, which can serve functions of advertising and patient recruitment. Online content can highlight the specialized features of an organization and be used to promote patient awareness. This will likely be important in a time of increasing transparency where surgical outcomes are publicly available [6]. This is especially true given recent data which suggests that the public may not be able to spot outliers in risk-adjusted data in order to better inform their healthcare decisions [7]. SMN may provide an opportunity for organizations to clarify the significance of outcome data. The use of SMN as a marketing tool for surgical practices has also been documented. In a 2013 survey of 500 members of the American Society of Plastic Surgeons, 50.4% reported the incorporation of SMN into their professional practice [8]. Use as a tool for effective marketing and patient education were among the most common reasons for utilization of SMN, and the majority of those surveyed felt it had positively impacted their practice. Notably, a significant proportion also felt more oversight was needed in order to uphold ethical standards.

Surgical colleges around the world are also utilizing SM in order to communicate with a greater audience and distribute information on a larger scale. An analysis of Twitter use by five prominent surgical colleges in the US and UK determined that these organizations have attained a significant international reach with their use of SM[9]. The content of posts was also included in the analysis and found to vary among the colleges. Those in the UK focused more on professional and educational development, while the American College of Surgeons (ACS) posted more content regarding patient outcomes. The ACS was the only surgical college with explicit plans regarding its goals for SM, which is to (1) promote the organization to prospective members and the public and (2) to enable interaction across the house of surgery [10]. The ACS has launched "ACS Communities", which is basically a social media platform where surgeons can exchange ideas, educate, collaborate, and optimize patient care in a protected online environment similar to closed Facebook groups. Having clearly defined SM policies may soon be considered best practice in order to focus online content.

SM usage for professional purposes by physicians has thus far been mostly through groups, profiles, or "pages" that are public, in which they can circulate publications, new research findings, or guidelines to patients and colleagues. However, more recently, physicians have been using the Facebook private groups feature or similar forums to engage in an online community of professionals in their field through discussion-based forums. These groups enable physicians to ask questions—either general, or about specific patient cases—to other physicians and provide a more private environment where the membership (and thus who can view or comment on posts) can be restricted.

Surgical practice, perhaps even more so than other specialties, engages in collaborative learning and quality improvement. Frequent morbidity and mortality conferences are perhaps the most notable form of this real-time peer review. However, not all surgeons work in practices with enough experienced surgeons to collaborate in person. With SM being increasingly used to facilitate discussion among a global community of surgeons, the scope of input a surgeon can receive regarding a particular case may increase exponentially. These types of forums can be particularly helpful for more rare conditions or complications which occur at a low frequency, since any individual physician may have little or no experience with a given issue, but drawing on the collective experience will help inform the best way to approach a rarer case.

The real-time nature of social media forums is perhaps one of the most valuable features for clinicians. The publication process in medicine is lengthy and time-consuming and ultimately causes significant delays between obtaining research results and disseminating findings to colleagues and then the general public. Additionally, in surgery in particular, the value of anecdotal evidence and personal experience cannot be denied, especially when referring to a complex case to which the results of carefully controlled clinical trials are not wholly generalizable. However, surgical journals tend to not focus on these types of information, although they can provide valuable insight to physicians in learning how to practically manage cases. Discussion of patient cases or general questions on SM forums may enable exchange of information more rapidly, without sacrificing the integrity of the peer-review process, since information can be disseminated instantaneously and discussion and questioning of anyone's information can ensue following the post. This peer-review process occurs on a much shorter time-scale than normal journal review, however, and may allow for discussions of more qualitative aspects of cases that don't necessarily fit into metrics commonly used in research.

Also important in advances in surgery are laboratory research, the technology and materials used to operate, and policies of hospitals and governing bodies in medicine. The exchange of ideas for research, changes in care models, different technique modifications, etc. can occur much more rapidly when information can be exchanged digitally and instantaneously from anywhere where there is an Internet connection. This information is able to cross hospital, regional, and national borders and broaden the perspectives of social media users greatly. Developing a framework of thinking that considers the opinions and practices of surgeons, scientists, and other medical professionals around the world may lead to new innovative solutions to problems that are generalizable and scalable to more than just one practice or hospital. Fostering an environment in which interdisciplinary collaboration can easily occur can contribute to increased cooperation between different branches of medicine and improvement in healthcare as a whole. Having an easy way to keep the lines of communication open between different spheres of medical research and care will make translational research and public health initiatives more in tune to what patients and physicians need and bring different perspectives together to create meaningful projects, policies, and products.

How Can SMN Benefit Patients?

When physicians are learning more about ways to improve their practice, patients are those who ultimately benefit. A means to engage physicians in a form of continuing medical education that they are enthusiastic about and voluntarily seek out will ultimately translate into continuous quality improvement that reflects in patient outcomes. Outside of the benefits patient glean from improved physician knowledge, there are additional ways SM can help patients manage their diseases and surgeries.

SM can be used to connect patients with resources to educate them about their disease or procedure. Social media is a sphere which, unlike medicine, most patients will feel comfortable navigating on their own due to personal experience with it on a daily basis. Breaking down barriers to health literacy by moving conversations about diseases and healthy lifestyles into an arena where patients feel they have more expertise and autonomy in the discussion can make them more engaged in their care. In an age where access to information online is rapidly changing the typical patient–physician encounter, doctors can help to guide patients to more informed decision-making by having social media resources at the ready to provide a reliable source for patients to learn more about their condition, rather than just searching through non-credible sources that may misinform or scare them. Physicians should be familiar with online information sources and social media resources for the diseases they treat, so that they can actively engage their patients and provide multiple channels for learning more about their conditions.

In addition to pure information, patients can read on social media about their illnesses, social media pages, and forums can recommend or provide tools to patients to help manage and keep track of symptoms, such as mobile apps or side effect journals. SM can also provide patients with support networks of others who suffer from similar conditions and information on local services available to a patient, such as discounted bus passes for handicapped patients. Social media can thus supplement medical treatment of a condition by helping address more of the social and emotional aspects of illness and helping patients feel more engaged in their health and treatment.

Maintaining Professionalism and Compliance

With the increase in SM usage among medical trainees and physicians comes concerns over professionalism. While SM provides the ability to share information quickly with a large audience, it also creates a lasting online record which often cannot be erased. Numerous cases of unprofessional behavior by medical students, resident, and practicing physicians have been memorialized online. For example, a recent nationwide assessment of surgical residents with publicly accessible Facebook accounts found that 14.1% had posted potentially unprofessional content and 12.2% had posted clearly unprofessional content [11]. The most commonly found offenses consisted of binge drinking, sexually suggestive photos, and Health Insurance Portability and Accountability Act (HIPAA) violations. The same assessment of attending surgeons yielded similar findings: 10.3% with potentially unprofessional content and 5.1% with clearly unprofessional content [12]. Such indiscretions have the potential to undermine the credibility of both individual surgeons and the medical profession as a whole.

In response to this need for professional self-regulation, the American Medical Association issued a report in 2011 which discusses the ethical implications of SM use by trainees and physicians [13]. It acknowledges that while SM use can support personal expression and foster professional collaboration, it also creates new challenges to the patient–physician relationship. The report offers several recommendations which are summarized as follows:

- Maintain standards of patient privacy.
- Liberal use of personal privacy settings with the realization that they are not infallible and that any content posted to the Internet is likely permanent.
- Any online communication with patients must be in-line with a professional patient–physician relationship.
- Separation of personal and professional content to help ensure professional boundaries.
- Taking action if witness to inappropriate content posted by colleagues. This may consist of notifying the offending colleague vs. an authority depending on the severity of the violation.
- Recognition that online content has the potential to harm one's own reputation and that of their colleagues and institution.

HIPAA regulations do state that patient case information can be shared outside of the patient's clinical care team if it is for the purposes of quality improvement. Although social media still falls into a "gray area" of the regulations given that it was not as prevalent when the law was written, many physicians believe that posting information about a de-identified patient case on social media is acceptable under HIPAA standards if it is for the purposes of either quality improvement and education or to consult other physicians for help managing the patient's treatment.

Posting information about a specific patient case to get advice or feedback for quality improvement when a complication occurs may be one of the most valuable ways to use social media and garner tips from professionals all over the world with different experiences. However, this type of situation offers the most potential for violations of patient privacy and HIPAA. To remain in compliance, physicians should at a minimum maintain the following standards for patient case posts:

- These should be restricted to private groups in which membership is monitored and controlled by a board of administrators. Members of the group ideally should also be held to a code of conduct in which they agree that any information they see posted in the group is for educational and quality improvement purposes only, or to help in that patient's treatment, and should not be disseminated in any way.
- All medical imaging, photos, or other content posted within the private group should be anonymized/de-identified. It should also be kept in mind that even though information such as name and date of birth may be removed from an image or video, patients with certain characteristics (very rare conditions, tumors, or hernias that have particularly unique features, very old age) may still be considered "identifiable" by HIPAA standards.
- Whenever possible, consent should be obtained from patients to share their case with a professional Facebook group. This should always be documented in writing if the case is being presented in a public forum, or if any identifying information will be included. For de-identified cases posted to professional private groups, consent may not be necessary but verbal consent at least is preferred. Patients will often appreciate a physician's desire to seek other opinions and input on the case and may even place more confidence in the management plan if their surgeon can present evidence to the patient that other experts agree with the course of treatment.

- If you are part of an institution, there will often be official policies regarding usage of social media by members of the institution. To avoid any potential violations and conflicts, these should be reviewed to make sure your practices are in line with the policies.

We believe surgeons who embrace social media platforms designed for quality improvement, with intent of continuing medical education or patient care optimization, should be protected from discoverability. That said, as of the writing of this manuscript, it is our belief that anything posted in a closed group or online community is subject to discoverability. We hope that should the situation arise, that the education gained from any post will help both the surgeon and the patient alike.

Specific Examples of SMN as a Tool in Surgical Practice

There are several examples of online collaborative engagements by surgeons. Some that exist on Facebook are: The International Bariatric Club, The Robotic Surgery Collaboration, SAGES Foregut Surgery Collaboration, and The International Hernia Collaboration (IHC). The International Hernia Collaboration (IHC) is a Facebook group established in December 2012 by Dr. Brian P. Jacob, which has grown into a community of hernia surgeons from around the world. The goal of the group is to facilitate discussion about all things related to hernias, to enable physicians to ask for advice, discuss the risks and benefits of different strategies and practices, debate the merits of new findings in the field, and disseminate information instantaneously to the global hernia surgery community. As a closed Facebook group, only vetted and approved members have access to create and view content. Additionally, posts are required to have any identifying information removed unless the patient has given express permission for their information to be shared with the forum. Posts that are unprofessional or that violate HIPAA compliance laws are deleted.

As of January 2017, membership has grown to 3100 members, with users being a mix of attending physicians, residents, medical students, and industry members. At any given day, there are over 500 surgeons in the vetting queue process, and an average of 4 to 6 new requests to join arrive daily. The administration is selective to admissions, with the goal being to optimize the quality and value of the discussion. Members represent over 63 different countries, with the vast majority of users being concentrated in the United States. Over the past year, there has been an average of 178 posts per month and 17 comments per post. There is a total of over 4300 posts in the forum, which can be searched with keywords by group members. Engagement is high, with 96% of posts being responded to, and both membership and group engagement have drastically increased since the creation of the group. These groups are a model for how SM can be used as a tool in continuing medical education, particularly by enabling interactive learning in real-time and providing access to the experience of experts in multiple subspecialties. The forum has direct applicability to clinical practice and patient outcome improvement, promotes awareness of differing resources and practices around the world, provides enhancement of research potential, and facilitates interdisciplinary collaboration.

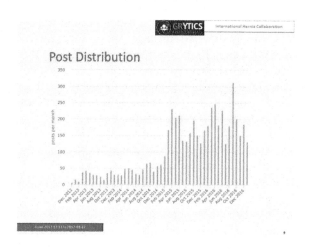

Summary guide for new surgeons establishing a digital foot-print online: when starting out, we recommend every surgeon consider buying a **website** domain name that defines the practice well. Hospital employees or large group employees will not need to do this as the hosptial or group will already have a website that they will add you to. If that hospital policy permits, it is always a good idea to still get your own website since many surgeons do move institutions throughout a career. This website should offer patient education, recovery information, and a way to contact the surgeon to promote dialogue. Next, surgeons should create at least one individual professional **Twitter** or **Facebook** account, and use it only for professional communication. Enrolling in an existing, or creating a new, closed Facebook **GROUP** or online specialty Community is a great way to collaborate and educate yourself and others within your specialty. In addition, your surgical practice can create a Facebook **PAGE** so that patients can interact with the business. Posting compliant videos on those sites or others like Youtube can be very beneficial to certain viewers. Use of other social media sites by surgeons, like SnapChat for example, continues to evolve, but we do not have enough experience to comment. Finally, you should check your **Google** status at least monthly. You will be automatically listed on rating websites like **HealthGrades and Vitals** (for example), but sites like **ZocDoc and Yelp** (for example) are paid by surgeons to keep a listing. All can be helpful, or hurtful. Learning how to manage all of those accounts is extremely important. Remember that you may move from hospital to hospital, but your online footprint will remain the same. Hundreds of patients will review you online in those sites, so you must review yourself often and learn how to contact those sites and optimize your presence on them.

Conclusion

Social media is a rapidly growing means of networking and communication among medical professionals, and has potential as a forum for discussion and education among surgeons and patients alike. While there are challenges to be faced regarding professionalism and privacy, the potential benefits far outweigh the negatives. We recommend that all surgeons, especially those new to practice, maintain an Internet presence that include the ways listed in Table 11.1. Surgeons should employ professional pages or profiles for their practice and/or themselves on several social media sites and also follow major academic and research organizations in their field on their respective pages. Maintaining a website with an independent domain name, where blogs and information for patients can be posted, is also highly recommended. As SM continues to make the world a smaller place, further opportunities for its use will surely present themselves. As surgeons, it is crucial that we remain innovators in this ever-changing technology.

TABLE 11.1 Social media and Internet usage recommendations for surgeons entering practice

New Surgeon guide to Internet presence	
Personal/Practice website	Unique domain name
	Blogs or testimonials
	Information for patients
Rating Website awareness	Yelp
	ZocDoc
	Vitals
	Healthgrades
	Google
Facebook	Member of a group or groups for your specialty
	Page for your patients and practice
Twitter	Professional handle for yourself (separate from personal handle)

References

1. Perrin A. Social networking usage: 2005–2015. Pew Research Center. October 2015.
2. Bosslet G, Torke A, Hickman S, et al. The patient–doctor relationship and online social networks: results of a national survey. J Gen Intern Med. 2012;26(10):1168–74.
3. Steele S, Arshad S, Bush R, et al. Social media is a necessary component of surgery practice. Surgery. 2015;158(3):857–62.
4. Maeve D, Ellison NB, Lampe C, Lenhart A, Madden M. Social Media Update 2014. Pew Research Center: Internet, Science & Tech. 2015 Jan 19; http://www.pewinternet.org/2015/01/09/social-media-update-2014/.
5. Crohnology. Web. 4 July 2016. http://www.crohnology.com.
6. Hospital Compare. Web. 4 July 2016. https://www.medicare.gov/hospitalcompare/
7. Bhalla A, Mehrotra P, Amawi F, et al. Surgeon-level reporting presented by funnel plot is understood by doctors but inaccurately interpreted by members of the public. J Surg Educ. 2015;72(3):500–3.
8. Vardanian A, Kusnezov N, Im D, et al. Social media use and impact on plastic surgery practice. Plast Reconstr Surg. 2013;131(5):1184–93.
9. Ralston M, O'Neill S, Wigmore S, et al. An exploration of the use of social media by surgical colleges. Int J Surg. 2014;12(12):1420–7.
10. Hoyt D. American College of Surgeons and social media efforts. Surgery. 2011;150(1):13–4.
11. Langenfeld S, Cook G, Sudbeck C, et al. An assessment of unprofessional behavior among surgical residents on Facebook: a warning of the dangers of social media. J Surg Educ. 2014;71(6):e28–32.
12. Langenfeld S, Sudbeck C, Luers T, et al. The glass houses of attending surgeons: an assessment of unprofessional behavior. J Surg Educ. 2014;71(6):e280–5.
13. Shore R, Halsey J, Shah K, et al. Report of the AMA Council on ethical and judicial affairs: professionalism in the use of social media. J Clin Ethics. 2011;22(2):165–72.

Part III

Chapter 12
Research: How to Set Up a Research Project

Maria S. Altieri and Aurora D. Pryor

Introduction

When you embark on a career in research, it is important to identify what you want to study, how to study it, what resources do you have (or need), and who will pay for it. This chapter will help you cover the basics. In terms of a research career, most surgeons find it helpful to pick areas for investigation that tie into topics they are interested in clinically or are directly related to issues they are working on, such as education paradigms. Resources at your institution or availability of mentors may help guide your research planning as well. Many junior surgeons start projects in several areas, but focus their careers in key areas based on their academic successes. This chapter will help you start in research from developing your first research project to securing funding.

M.S. Altieri, M.D.
Department of Surgery, Stony Brook University Medical Center, Stony Brook, NY, USA

A.D. Pryor, M.D. (✉)
Division of Bariatric, Foregut, and Advanced Gastrointestinal Surgery, Department of Surgery, Health Sciences Center T18-040, Stony Brook Medicine, Stony Brook, NY 11794-8191, USA
e-mail: aurora.pryor@stonybrookmedicine.edu

© Springer International Publishing AG 2017
D.B. Renton et al. (eds.), *The SAGES Manual Transitioning to Practice*, DOI 10.1007/978-3-319-51397-3_12

Identifying a Topic and Developing a Research Question

Developing a research question and a topic is the first step towards starting a project. Topics should be carefully selected, clearly defined, and focused. In addition, they should involve a specific unique area or area where deficits exist. The research question and specific aims should help guide and focus the study. Prior to developing a research question, it is important to ensure that previous investigations are not duplicated by performing an extensive literature search [1]. Typical search engines include PubMed, Web of Science, Scopus, Enbase, Clinicaltrials.gov, Cinahl, Cochrane Database. These search engines can help you figure out if the specific question is already published. In addition, you can search the conference proceedings to confirm that your research question has also not been previously presented. If presented at a conference, you should suspect that a publication is in process.

If any relevant research has been performed, these studies should be carefully reviewed to examine if any deficits or inconsistencies exist, which can be expanded upon by you. Based on this review, your question can be modified to include a different aspect of the topic. If the published research is relatively weak (small sample size, short period of follow-up, or not an appropriate control study population), a better study can be designed to improve on the weakness of previously published work. A thorough background review is critical to establish a research question, as the main goal of research is to study something novel or improve on previously done research so that you can present your work and be published.

It is important to have a mentor or study collaborator that has a strong background/expertise in the area of interest. Since the most important part of designing a research question is the initial work, establishing an early collaboration is vital. An expert can help hone in on specific areas of deficits

TABLE 12.1 PICO method

P	Population/patient
I	Intervention
C	Comparator, control
O	Outcome

and help guide the study design and methodology. Ideally, this collaboration will be within the same institution or department. In case there are no experts in the area of research at your institution, you can seek an outside collaboration. Frequent meetings/conference calls regarding progress in the study are essential.

Next, it is important to refine the question and establish the study aims or objectives [1, 2]. A systematic way to refine your research question is to use the PICO method. The PICO method is described in Table 12.1. You can use the PICO method as the pillars for establishing the study protocol.

Study Protocol

The study protocol is the blueprint of the study. A typical protocol involves several sections, including: Background, Objectives/Specific Aims, Preliminary Studies, Research Design and Methods, Statistical Design and Analysis, Funding Status/Budget, Data Safety Monitoring Plan, Risks and Benefit to participants, Confidentiality to participants, and Milestones. This document should encompass everything about the study and should be used as a guide to the researcher through the study. A simple study such as a chart review will have a shorter study protocol, compared to a randomized control trial, which ideally should include every detail regarding the study. Clinical trials are governed by the ICH Good Clinical Practice Guidelines, as they describe the responsibilities and expectations of all participants in the conduct of clinical trials [3]. Table 12.2 shows the topics of a

TABLE 12.2 A sample protocol based on ICH good clinical practice guidelines

- Title page/general information
- Background information
- Trial objectives/purpose
- Study design
- Selection and withdrawal of subjects
- Treatment of subjects
- Assessment of efficacy
- Assessment of safety
- Statistics
- Direct access to source data and documents
- Quality control and assurance
- Ethics
- Data handling and record keeping
- Financing and insurance
- Publication policy
- Supplements/appendices

protocol as outlined by the ICH Good Clinical Practice. NIH and other organizations use this template for grant applications. However, others have mandatory requirements for using a specific protocol.

Based on the type of study, research may need approval prior to initiation. If the study involves reviews of the literature or meta-analyses, there is no need for prior approval.

However, if there is a direct interaction with patients/subjects/ animals, permission from the Institutional Review Board (IRB) or the Institutional Animal Care and Use Committee (IACUC) may be necessary prior to study implementation. For further information, please see the later section.

What Resources Will You Need to Be Successful?

The success of research will be determined not only by the topic, but also at the resources available. Research takes time and commitment. Balancing between clinical responsi- bilities and conducting research may prove a challenge. Based on your practice setting, you may have different resources at your disposal. Funding may also play an impor- tant role. Funding can be obtained from institutional funds or grants from government, society, or industry. In addition, research support in the form of research assistants, co- investigators, consultants, and statisticians may be needed. Such resources are more often available in the academic setting.

IRB and IACUC

Research involving humans and animals must be done with accordance with ethical principles and policies. Institutional Review Board (IRB) and Institutional Animal Care and Use Committee (IACUC) are two institutional committees whose purpose is to assure sound research.

Under governmental regulation, an IRB is a group of researchers and physicians who are designated to review and monitor biomedical research involving human subjects. This group, which is institutionally based, has the authority to approve, modify, or disapprove research. If an institution does not have an internal IRB, the institution can arrange for an outside IRB to review and oversee the studies. The IRB usually meets on timed intervals during which they review research applications, protocols, and related materials, such as consents, brochures and recruitment materials, data collection sheets, questionnaires, package inserts for approved drugs/devices, in order to ensure protection of the rights and welfare of human subjects. For information regarding process, every institution conducting research has a central resource, typically a website, which has comprehensive explanations regarding the paperwork and committee policies. Prior to applying, the individuals involved should be trained in human subjects training. Our institution is a subscriber to the web-based CITI training program, which contains modules for Human Subjects, Animal Use, Stem Cells, Conflict of Interest, Responsible Conduct of Research and Scholarship (RCRS) training in various academic disciplines. The training in human subjects includes HIPAA and human subjects protection training. For specific requirements, please refer to the office of research compliance at your institution.

There are usually three types of applications, depending on the project: Exemption, Expedited, and Full review. Exempt studies involve research on human subjects per federal definition, but falls into one of the six exempt categories. Table 12.3 describes the six classifications [4]. Exempt studies do not require IRB approval. However, most institutions have their IRB review all protocols and make the exempt determination [5]. Expedited review involves research on subjects and requires review, but does not require a full review by the IRB committee, as it poses no more than minimal risk to subjects. Retrospective study involving chart review is an example of a study necessitating an expedited review. Full review is required where more than minimal risk is anticipated. Such studies usually involve randomized controlled trials. For a new investigator, it's a good idea to find a contact at your IRB and ask for direction on your submissions. It is good form even for projects that do not require IRB

TABLE 12.3 Exempt studies

101 (b)(1):	**Research conducted in established or commonly accepted educational settings, involving normal educational practices**
101 (b)(2)	Research involving the use of educational tests (cognitive, diagnostic, aptitude, achievement), survey procedures, interview procedures, or observation of public behavior, unless both of the following are true: 1. Subjects can be identified directly or indirectly AND 2. Any disclosure of the human subjects' responses outside the research could reasonably place the subjects at risk of criminal or civil liability or be damaging to the subjects' financial standing, employability, or reputation 3. This category does not apply to any research involving minors
101 (b)(3)	Research involving the use of educational tests (cognitive, diagnostic, aptitude, achievement), surveys, interviews, or observation of public behavior that is not exempt under paragraph (b)(2) above, if subjects are elected or appointed public officials or candidates
101 (b)(4)	Research involving existing data (documents, specimens, etc.) if 1. These sources are publicly available, OR 2. If the information is de-identified
101 (b)(5)	Research and demonstration projects conducted or approved by a federal agency head, and which are designed to study any of the following: 1. Public benefit or service programs 2. Procedures for obtaining benefits or services under those programs 3. Possible changes in those programs; or 4. Possible changes in methods or levels of payment for benefits under those programs
101 (b)(6)	Taste and food quality evaluation and consumer acceptance studies

approval to get an email back from the IRB confirming that review is not required.

The Institutional Animal Care and Use Committee (IACUC) is of central importance to the governing of animal research. The IACUC committee is responsible for reviewing all studies involving vertebrate animals and ensuring training and compliance involving animals, in addition to assuring animal facilities and laboratories are up to date with regulations. Training for animal research is more intense as investigators need to have animal husbandry and management experience. Requirements can include occupational health clearance, completion of specific training modules, reviewing standard procedures of the facility, reviewing federal compliance regulations, and an introductory course by the animal facility. For requirements specific to your institution, please contact your research compliance office.

The application typically requires a detailed protocol, consent (when appropriate), and several application forms specific for the type of review and for the institution. The Research Compliance Office at the associated institution is a great resource for any IRB- or IACUC-related questions.

Sources of Funding

There are several sources of funding, such as university grants, government agencies (NIH), industry, and surgical societies. The amount of funding is variable as university grants and surgical societies have more limited funding compared to government agencies- and industry-sponsored research. Certain hospitals and departments will offer grant opportunities to encourage research. For information or availability of such grants, contact the department of research at your institution. These internal funds are usually the first place to start for seed funds or for new investigators. Negotiation for these funds can even be part of your initial contract discussion.

Industry funding can be either industry-initiated or investigator-initiated. In some instances, industry will contact an investigator/institution for a participation in a study, such as a clinical trial. This type of research support is usually straightforward for junior investigators to obtain and is typically the first source of funding outside of your own institution. Most industry support is received as investigator-initiated studies (IIS). Many pharmaceutical or device companies have adopted this process. In an IIS, the investigator is responsible for all facets of the study, including concept and protocol development, budget development, ethic and IRB submission, and trial management. Usually, these studies involve already approved drugs or devices. The process involves several steps, starting with the principal investigator submitting an application to the sponsor, including a detailed protocol, budget, approval by the institution, and any other information required by the sponsor. The sponsor will review the proposal and can negotiate terms and conditions. If both parties are in agreement, the sponsor will execute a contract and establish an award. Examples of IIS sponsors and links to websites are provided in Table 12.4.

Another example of collaboration between industry and an investigator is in the form of an industry-initiated trial. Usually, the goal of such partnership is to develop a new

TABLE 12.4 Examples of companies involved in investigator-initiated studies

Covidien	http://www.covidien.com/investigatorsponsoredresearch/
Ethicon	https://www.ethicon.com/corporate/our-connections/other-funding/investigator-initiated-studies
Bard-Davol	http://www.davol.com/clinical-support/iss/
Cook Medical	https://www.cookmedical.com/charitable-donations-grants-sponsorships/guidelines/
Medtronic	http://professional.medtronic.com/customer-support/research-proposal-contacts/#Vln8vGSrSCQ

product or gain FDA approval of a new drug or product. The company will provide the funding and expect intellectual property rights or results from the research. The sponsor may be responsible for compliance with ICH Good Clinical Practice, Protocol design, Standard of Operative Procedures, and availability of appropriate staff and facilities in order to conduct research.

Surgical Societies are another great source of funding. This type of funding is usually appropriate when you have a solid idea and some research experience. Societies will announce the opportunity for application to their members, usually on an annual basis. The grants will vary based on the purpose of the society. For example, the Society of American Gastrointestinal and Endoscopic Surgeons (SAGES) offers SAGES Research Grants, Fundamentals Use of Surgical Energy™ Grants, Fundamentals of Endoscopic Surgery™ Grants, SAGES SMART™ Enhanced Recovery Grants, in addition to a Career Development Award. Surgical society grants are usually competitive, but are great for small projects. Some of these societies will encourage grant funding to young investigators and those that are involved in the society. The application forms and requirements are usually displayed on the internet. Society funding is a good way to establish a successful funding track record and build up your CV for future government funding.

National Institute of Health Awards: What Are They and Who Are They for?

The National Institutes of Health (NIH) is the nation's primary agency of the United States government, which is responsible for funding and conducting biomedical research. It is comprised of 27 separate institutes and centers. The NIH both conducts and also provides major biomedical research funding to others through its extramural research program. The NIH provides many different types of grants, several of which will be described here.

Career Development Awards

The NIH has a long-standing history of supporting physicians in terms of providing funding, salary, mentorship, and protected time. Between 1957 and 2011, the NIH has provided more than 19,000 career development awards, also known as "K awards", at a total cost of over $8 billion [6]. There are nine different career development awards that physicians can consider. Information regarding these awards can be accessed on https://researchtraining.nih.gov/programs/career-development. Most of these awards are intended for physicians who have completed their training and have a faculty position. Some of the career development awards are institution-specific, such as the Mentored Clinical Scientist Developmental Program Award (K12). Others are individual awards, such as the Mentored Research Scientist Development Award (K01), the Mentored Clinical Scientist Development Award (K08), or the Mentored Patient-Oriented Research Career Development Award (K23). Most applicants to the K01 awards are PhDs, while most applicants for K08 and K23 awards are MDs or MD/PhDs. In addition, the mid-career Investigator Award in Patient-Oriented Research (K24) allows for an already established surgeon to mentor junior clinicians.

Mentored Clinical Scientist Development Award (K08)

Purpose

The purpose of this award is to provide support and protected time for individuals with a health-professional doctoral degree for an intensive, supervised research career development experience in the fields of biomedical and behavioral research for a span of 3–5 years.

General Information

There were 3751 awards between FY 1990-FY 2005 and 7754 applicants during the same time period with a 48% award rate [6]. These awards are targeted for people in a postdoctorate/residency or early career. The applicant must be a US citizen or permanent resident and must have a clinical doctoral degree, either M.D., D.O., or equivalent. At least 2 years must have elapsed since the degree was obtained. In addition, the applicant must have a professional license to practice in the US.

The candidate must obtain the mentorship of a senior physician, who can provide guidance in the specific area of interest. Institutions can submit applications on behalf of candidates and it must show that they have the staff and facilities needed for the proposed research. The applicant must spend at least nine person-months (75% of full-time professional effort), conducting research and related career development activities.

Mentored Patient-Oriented Research Career Development Award (K23)

Purpose

The purpose of a K23 award is to provide support and "protected time" to non-tenured investigators interested in mentored patient-oriented research. Candidates must have a clinical degree and practice.

General Information

There were 1249 awards between FY 2000- FY 2005 and 3083 applicants with an award rate of 41% [1]. Similar to K08 awards, the K23 award provides support for a 3–5 year period.

Candidates for this award must have completed their training and be willing to spend a minimum of 75% of full-time professional effort conducting research.

R Grants

There are several types of research ("R") grants, as this chapter will describe the NIH Small Grant (R03), Exploratory/development grants (R21), and NIH research project grant (R01).

Small Grant (R03)

The small grant is intended to support small research project that can be carried out with limited resources in a short period of time. The grant provides up to $50,000 and covers up to 2 years of research time. This grant cannot be renewed and it allows for one resubmission. It does not require preliminary data. It is intended for pilot or feasibility studies, small research projects, development of research methodology or new technology, or analysis of existing data [7]. Please check with the specific NIH institute, as not all institutes provide small grants.

Exploratory/Development Research Grants (R21)

Exploratory/Developmental research grants provide funding for novel ideas, model systems, tools, and technologies that have the potential to advance biomedical research. No preliminary data is required; however, most investigators provide such data. These grants fund up to 2 years of support and up to $275,000. Like R03 grants, they are not renewable and not all institutes provide these grants. Some investigators use these grants to obtain preliminary results in order to apply for R01 grants.

NIH Research Project (R01)

Research Project Grants (R01) is the most common source of funding for investigators and can help establish one's research career. These grants are the most competitive grants, as they provide funding support for up to 5 years and budgets up to $500,000 per year in direct costs, although higher amounts can be requested. The grant application requires preliminary data.

For more information about research grants, please visit the NIH website: http://grants.nih.gov/grants/about_grants.htm.

Other Funding Sources:

In addition to the funding sources mentioned above, many investigators have had successful experiences with other government agencies such as the Patient-Centered Outcomes Research Institute (PCORI) or Department of Defense. There is also funding available through many philanthropic organizations, such as the Roberts Woods Johnson Foundation. Many of these groups can be identified by discussions with your mentors or by collaboration with other investigators.

Summary

There are many great opportunities for surgical research. We hope these resources help you find a topic that is interesting and start the framework for a successful career.

References

1. Hanson PB. Designing, conducting, and reporting clinical research: a step-by-step approach. Injury. 2006;37:538–94.
2. Grover FL, Shroyer AL. Clinical science research. J Thorac Cardiovasc Surg. 2000;119(4 Pt 2):S11–21.

3. International Conference on Harmonisation of Technical Requirements for Registration of Pharmaceuticals for Human Use. Guideline for Good Clinical Practice E6 (R1). 1996. Accessed November 11, 2015 at http://www.ich.org/products/guidelines/efficacy/efficacy-single/article/good-clinical-practice.html.

4. United States Department of Health and Human Services, Code for Federal Regulations. Protection of Human Subjects (Part 46). 2009. Accessed October 23, 2015 at http://www.hhs.gov/ohrp/humansubjects/guidance/45cfr46.html.

5. United States Department of Health and Human Services, ORRP Reports. Exempt Research and research that may undergo expedited review. 1995. Accessed November 11, 2015 at http://www.hhs.gov/ohrp/policy/hsdc95-02.html.

6. National Institutes of Health Individual Mentored Career Development Awards Program Evaluation Working Group, National Institutes of Health Individual Mentored Career Development Awards Program. Accessed August 29, 2015 at http://grants.nih.gov/training/K_awards_evaluation_finalReport_20110901.pdf, 2011.

7. United States Department of Health and Human Services. National Institutes of Health, Office of Extramural Research. Grants and Funding. Accessed November 23, 2015 at http://grants.nih.gov/grants/funding/r03.htm.

Chapter 13
Manuscript Writing

Pritam Singh and Rajesh Aggarwal

Where to Start?

Surgeons can be great procrastinators when it comes to writing a scientific manuscript. This is often borne out of a combination of fear and dislike of writing paragraphs when surgeons are used to writing short sharp factual comments. One method to alleviate this is to bullet point the content you wish to put in the manuscript. This gets words on the page and avoids the despair of staring at a blank page. People will have different advice on which section to start with, but in general it is often easiest to start by writing the methods and results. These are factual sections with minimal interpretation required. While the introduction and conclusion should also be based on facts, they allow and require a certain amount of interpretation in order to make them interesting and of value.

P. Singh, M.B.B.S., M.A., M.R.C.S.
Division of Surgery, Department of Surgery & Cancer, Imperial College London & West Midlands Deanery, London, UK

R. Aggarwal, M.B.B.S., M.A., Ph.D., F.R.C.S. (✉)
Department of Surgery, Faculty of Medicine, McGill University, 3575 Parc Avenue, Suite 5640, Montreal, Quebec, Canada
e-mail: rajesh.aggarwal@mcgill.ca

Steinberg Centre for Simulation and Interactive Learning, Faculty of Medicine, McGill University, Montreal, Quebec, Canada

© Springer International Publishing AG 2017   189
D.B. Renton et al. (eds.), *The SAGES Manual Transitioning to Practice*, DOI 10.1007/978-3-319-51397-3_13

Reading other journal articles will help you develop a writing style. Furthermore, you will need to read and be cognizant of the literature relevant to your study being reported. If there are certain research groups or authors whose work is prominent in your field of study, then remember that they may well be chosen by the journal to review your manuscript. This chapter provides information for the early stage researcher. The guidelines are not absolute and you will develop your own writing style and preferences as you become more experienced. You may even alter your style to meet the audience or the message you are trying to get across. You will also likely change your writing style based on the type of manuscript you are preparing.

Types of Manuscript

There are many different types of articles and it is important to both be familiar with the different types and be aware of which type of manuscript you are writing as they will often require different writing styles. These include

- Original articles
- Editorials
- Commentaries
- Letters

While letters, commentaries, or editorials can be invited articles, original articles are usually peer-reviewed and this is what this chapter will focus on. Within original articles, there are some specific subtypes:

- Meta-analysis of Randomised Controlled Trials
- Randomised Controlled Trials
- Systematic Reviews
- Case-control studies
- Case-series

Some of these study types have well-established guidelines regarding reporting standards. For meta-analyses, these include the MOOSE [1] (Meta-Analysis Of Observational

Studies in Epidemiology) guidelines, the PRISMA [2] (Preferred Reporting Items for Systematic reviews and Meta-Analyses) statement, and the STROBE [3] (Strengthening the Reporting of Observational Studies in Epidemiology) statement. The PRISMA guidelines appear to be the most popular in the published literature, but it is worth being familiar with all of them. For randomized controlled trials, the CONSORT [4] (Consolidated Standards of Reporting Trials) statement is a valuable resource.

Links to:

MOOSE: http://www.ncbi.nlm.nih.gov/ pubmed/10789670, http://jama.jamanetwork.com/article. aspx?articleid=192614

PRISMA: http://www.ncbi.nlm.nih.gov/ pubmed/19622511,   http://annals.org/article. aspx?articleid=744664

STROBE: http://www.strobe-statement.org/

CONSORT: http://www.consort-statement.org/

Practical Tips

Reference Managers and Journal Styles

Once you start to write the introduction and discussion sections, you will need to refer to the relevant literature. This is essential, but can be time consuming if you try to do this manually, as each time you add a reference, you will have to amend your bibliography and update all the citation numbers in the text. Investing some time getting familiar with and using a reference manager program will save a lot of time at a later date. Some examples of reference management programs include:

- Papers (Mekentosj B.V. Van Godewijckstraat, Amsterdam, The Netherlands)
- Endnote (Thomson Reuters, New York, USA)
- Mendeley (Mendeley, Inc., New York, USA)

Word Processing

Whichever word processing programs you use, become familiar with its functions and make use of these features. The key is to minimize the need to procrastinate. While the words are flowing, if there is something you are unsure of such as the exact reference or the cost of something etc., rather than breaking the flow of your writing and searching for this detail, use the 'add note' function and come back to the detail at a later time. Notes can then be detailed at a later date when you are finalizing the first draft.

Similarly when reviewing the paper, you can also add notes which can be useful for yourself and your co-authors when they come to review the draft manuscript. Save your work regularly and in a logical order. Some tables or figures can slow down the main file, e.g. when loading the file or scrolling up and down. It may be better to not include them in the main manuscript and to keep tables and figures backed up in separate files to the main manuscript. This is the way in which most journals will ask for the manuscript to be submitted, so it is an efficient way to work.

If there are multiple authors simultaneously working on a paper, make sure you have an accurate and logical mechanism of tracking which version each author is working on. Using the 'track changes' function can allow multiple authors to easily make simultaneous changes and then send it back to the main author. This reduces the problems with authors using older versions as any changes can be easily identified. A software program that allows multiple authors to edit the same file could also be used such as Google Docs (Google, Inc. California, USA).

Which Journal to Submit to?

This stage is after the manuscript is complete, but where possible it is better to consider the journal before you start writing. When choosing your journal, consider the correct audience for your work and compare that with the readership of your potential journal. A high impact journal is desirable, but you may find that the readership is broad. Specialist journals may target the readership you are after, but this may come at the expense of impact factor. Be realistic about the impact of the work you are submitting. It is good to aim high, but early or pilot observational data may not be suitable for high impact journals until further data is obtained from the larger planned study. Read articles in the journals you plan to submit to in order to gain insight as to whether your manuscript is the kind of work they publish. Consider the work you plan to cite in your own manuscript and where that has been published.

Once a journal has been selected, take time to read the 'instructions for authors'. These will contain practical advice in terms of the formatting:

- Preferred reference style to be used in the bibliography and how to present the citation throughout the manuscript.

  - Remember you can usually download these reference styles directly to your reference manager to save manually updating the reference manager settings.

- The subheadings for the manuscript will be explained.
- Restrictions on words, pages, number of tables, and figures will be stated.

Tailor your manuscript to the audience who tend to read the journal. For instance, 'Surgical Endoscopy' readers will likely be laparoscopic surgeons, while 'Annals of Surgery' readers are likely to be cardiovascular and ENT surgeons, for example, in addition to the surgical endoscopy readers. A broad medical journal such as the Lancet or the New England Journal of Medicine will include non-surgical readers, so bear this in mind when writing the manuscript and in particular when describing the technicalities of the surgical techniques.

Writing the Content

Title

The importance of the title is often underestimated. When your manuscript is published and a PAP alert (Published Ahead of Print) or an eTOC alert (email with the table of contents for the next issue of a journal) is sent out, the title is often the only piece of information the potential reader will see. Therefore, it must instantly engage the potential reader to proceed and read the abstract. There is a fine balance between a descriptive and serious title versus interesting or controversial titles. Your choice may change depending on what you are hoping to achieve. You may be trying to court controversy, but remember this is a riskier approach as the reviewers may not be appreciative of this style. Our advice would be to start with a conservative classic and informative title. Once the manuscript is completed, you may wish to be bolder with the title. The title should make clear the question investigated and the study design, particularly if you have a strong study design such as a randomized controlled trial.

Methods

This should be the most straightforward section to write and is often a good section to get started with. If you have submitted an ethics application or applied for a grant, then the chances are that you have already written most of this already and it may only need tweaking. To the clinician scientist, this is probably the most important section of the manuscript as the results, and any interpretation of them, are only valid if the methods are robust. It is your role as the author to demonstrate all the steps taken to ensure the methods are valid and reliable and the steps you have taken to reduce the bias in the study. If a particular sample size was chosen for the study, then the rationale behind this should be explained.

This would be strengthened if a formal power calculation had been performed and this should be included in the methods section if it was. You need to carefully describe the study design, so it is clear and unambiguous. A scientist in a similar field of work as yourself should be able to glean enough information from your methods section to repeat the studies you have conducted. There clearly needs to be a balance between important detail and maintaining the reader's interest. Remember, if there are lengthy fine details required to replicate your work, these can be referred to in an appendix. If the reviewers deem these to be important, many journals will upload these as supplementary online material. Also remember that if the methods have been used by your group in previously published work or if the methods themselves have been previously published, you can simply cite these references in order to shorten the length of your own manuscript.

For certain types of articles, there are established guidelines on how they should be reported. You should be familiar with these and refer to them if appropriate:

- Randomised Controlled Trials—CONSORT [4] guidelines.
- Meta-analyses—MOOSE [1], PRISMA [2], or STROBE [3] guidelines.

Diagrams can often be useful in order to demonstrate the flow of subjects within the study. A CONSORT diagram is essential for randomized controlled trials. A well-written methods section will include details of the analyses planned. This should make clear the outcomes that will be measured. The study's primary outcome and secondary outcomes should be explicitly stated. The planned statistical analyses including the test that will be used and the level of significance chosen should be stated together with details of the statistical software to be used. Be prepared to defend your choice of statistical analysis if the reviewers ask for this. If in doubt, and where possible, seek guidance from a professional statistician. While this is the ideal, professional statisticians may not be easily accessible, particularly to the early stage researcher. Most clinicians will know a 'go-to' person within their Department who may well be a clinician, but is also well-versed in statistical analysis. Often the statistics required are not difficult and are fairly commonly used unless you have a complex study design. It is therefore useful to use these opportunities to build your own statistical knowledge by seeking guidance rather than delegating the analysis out to a third party.

Results

This section should clearly and concisely state the outcomes you set out to measure. It may seem obvious, but remember this section is a statement of the facts. The results section is not the place to try and interpret or explain the outcomes measured; this should be left to the discussion. This should therefore make the results section straightforward to write and this is why it is a good section to write straight after the methods section. The results should be presented in the manner in which the study was planned in the methods section. This means that the primary outcomes should be the mainstay of the results section. If the secondary outcomes are more interesting or surprising, it is reasonable to report them, but remember the study will have been designed and perhaps powered to assess the primary outcome rather than the secondary outcomes and this is what the reader will be most interested in.

The results section should contain all the statistical analyses including all the p values. Be consistent with your results reporting, choose the number of significant figure or decimal places you report to and maintain it. The number chosen should be stated explicitly either in the results or the methods section. Tables and graphs that can convey more data in fewer words are a good idea. However, they should not be included if they simply repeat the information in the text. Journals will often charge for colour images, so bear this in mind when designing your graphs or if you plan to include illustrations. You may wish to use hatched bars instead of colours for your charts, if you do not intend to pay the extra supplement for colour images. Furthermore, journals have restrictions on the number of tables and figures they allow, so it is worth looking into this if you expect to have more than two or three. Take care in formatting the tables and graphs; they should be visually appealing, but more importantly they must be clear and easy to interpret. If the table or figure is complex or something that is not commonly used, then use the figure legends to assist the reader to interpret the information.

Introduction

Once you have written the methods and results section, you should be getting into the flow of writing and will be better placed to write the introduction. The key in the introduction is to convince the reader that your work is not only interesting, but it is essential! Ideally, the reader should finish reading the introduction thinking 'why has nobody done this before'. Some background information is needed, but the introduction should not be too lengthy, as this may bore the reader. There is a tendency for the introduction to start with a very broad opening paragraph. While this may be appropriate for some instances, particularly when it is a niche subject area, often the first paragraph can be tightened up when you return to it after the manuscript is complete.

Approximately, three paragraphs should be appropriate for most manuscripts. It is worth citing some key studies, but the majority of the literature review can be left for the discussion. The level of detail required in the background will very much depend on the audience you are writing for. The readership of NEJM will include non-surgeons, whereas the readership of Surgical Endoscopy are likely to be surgeons with a laparoscopic interest. The final paragraph should make clear the study question that you are seeking to answer. This will provide a good lead into the methods section and the reader then knows what to expect from the rest of the manuscript. If the question is vague, the reader may lose interest.

Discussion

This is probably the most difficult section to write as it requires both a detailed understanding of your results and also an appreciation of how this fits into the relevant literature. That said, it can also be the most rewarding section to write as it is your opportunity to convey to the reader the potential impact of your endeavors. The key objective of the discussion is to facilitate the reader in answering the following question:

- What is the novel contribution of your work to the literature?

The section should summarize the key and important results and then go on to offer an interpretation of them. Remember you have already given the detailed figures with p values in the results section, so you should summarize the general trends found rather than repeat your results section.

Include any salient limitations and alternative explanations for your results. If you can think of a limitation, so will the reviewers. Therefore, it is preferable to make it clear that you have already identified these limitations and perhaps offer an explanation of how they could be improved if possible. Similarly, if there are alternative interpretations or explanations for your results, the reviewer is likely to identify this. You should offer these interpretations and then explain, based on your results, why you think your interpretation is the most accurate. Remember the limitations do not need to be exhaustive, just the salient points will suffice. It is good to end the discussion on a positive note, so following the limitations it would be useful to discuss future work. It is likely that further study will be required to confirm your interpretation, so you can explain how you intend to do this; you may even be conducting these studies at the time.

Conclusion

Not all journals require a separate conclusion; if they do not, then it is still worth having a concluding paragraph. Once again, use this section to highlight what your novel contribution to the literature is. Did you answer the hypothesis or question you asked at the start of the study? What are the implications of your work? Try not to overstate your conclusion as this will irritate reviewers, but you do need to make clear what the take home message of your manuscript is.

Abstract

This is the only part of the manuscript the majority of people will read. Therefore, it needs to be engaging enough to encourage the reader to read the whole manuscript and must include the key take home message of the work. A good abstract will encourage a reader to read a manuscript they may only have an outside interest in. Often a manuscript is written after the study has been presented at a scientific conference and an abstract is already available before the manuscript has been written. This initial abstract can be used as a starting point, but ensure you look at it in detail and revise it if necessary. You may have collected more data since your presentation, so the results will need to be updated. After the feedback received during your presentation, you may find yourself adapt your take home message—for instance you may need to avoid overstating it.

If you do not already have an abstract, then it is often best to write it at the end. Abstracts are usually limited to between 250 to 400 words, so you need to be fairly ruthless in what you can include. You will not be able to fit in all the results, but you must include the primary outcomes and anything else that is interesting should take priority over a long list of negatives.

Abstracts are generally structured similar to the manuscript. Keep the introduction succinct as there will not be enough words to explain the whole background. Focus on the methods and results, as this is what people will scrutinize. This is your place to demonstrate a robust study design, so make study design and make sure keywords are included such as:

- Randomised
- Prospective
- Controlled
- Blinded

State the take home message in the conclusion.

After Submission of the Manuscript

You can feel proud of reaching this stage, which is an achievement in itself, but this is the time to focus and ensure you do not lose momentum. There will be one of three outcomes at this stage:

Acceptance This is very unlikely, almost all editors will request at least one round of corrections before accepting a paper.

Revisions requested This is generally the best-case scenario. The editors and reviewers essentially like your work, but if your corrections are not comprehensive then they can still reject your work

Rejection This is often hard to take, particularly if the reviewers have been a bit brutal with their assessment of your work. However, if you aim high, this is an inevitability at some stage and the key is to use the editor's and the reviewers' comments constructively in order to enhance your manuscript and submit it to another journal.

How to Respond to Rejection

Do not take it personally. It can be hard to see your hard work criticized; however, this is not the time to get defensive as there is generally no ulterior motive to the rejection other than it was not suitable for the journal for one of many reasons. Occasionally, if you feel the review process has been unduly biased, then you can write to the journal editor with some thoughts. This is not advisable for the vast majority of rejections and it would not be recommended without prior consultation and advice from a senior researcher first.

There can be many reasons for a rejection. The editor may have felt the manuscript was not suited to their audience. This is probably the easiest rejection to deal with and is not uncommon. In the quest for high impact publications, we can be encouraged to submit to very broad based journals whose readers will only be interested in the manuscript if it really is practice changing. Have an honest look at your manuscript and choose another journal taking on board the editors' comments.

If you have received comments by reviewers, then go through them in detail and try to use the feedback to improve the manuscript and resubmit to another journal after considering where would be best to submit. A *good* rejection will give you plenty of constructive comments to work on and you can really strengthen your manuscript. Remember, unlike when you have been invited to submit a revision, you do not necessarily need to respond to every comment if you feel strongly that it will not improve your manuscript.

How to Respond to Corrections

As outright acceptance of a manuscript is vanishingly rare, in general being invited to respond to reviewers' comments is a successful outcome. Minor corrections are usually self-explanatory and can be fairly simple to make, so you can be hopeful that the manuscript will be accepted. Major corrections can vary in their detail and may even require some further analyses. For this reason, they can and do still get rejected if you are not careful in your response. There are some key steps that still need to be taken regardless of how extensive the corrections requested are. A cover letter should be written outlining that you have responded to each and every comment or question by the reviewers. One way to do this is to have a separate 'response to reviewer comments' document, which has the reviewer comments copied and pasted in it. After each comment or question, make a response and include any sections of the manuscript that have been changed along with the page and lines in the revised manuscript where these changes can be found. Essentially, you want to make it as easy as possible for the reviewers to see and identify how you have responded to their questions.

It is crucial to address all comments and questions the reviewer has made. This does not mean you have to accept all their suggestions; in fact some suggestions may not be possible to correct or may be contradictory to what one of the other reviewers suggest. Occasionally, you may simply disagree with the reviewer's comment or suggestion. However, even if you do not make a change to the manuscript, you must provide a response to demonstrate that you have considered their opinion. The revisions to your manuscript can be made while using the 'track changes' function on your word processor. Some journals will invite you to submit the revised article with the 'tracked changes' visible, while others will not, but in any case it will be useful for you and your co-authors to have the changes visible to ensure you have responded appropriately.

Your Manuscript Is Accepted: What Next?

Now you can allow yourself and your co-authors to celebrate. In due course, you will be sent proofs and may even be asked to respond to some letters about your article. The proofs deserve your attention as you may find that, in the formatting for a journal, some errors have crept in. Ensure the references are correct, particularly their order, and websites addresses. The manuscript acceptance process from submission to final publication can take up to 6 months or even a year depending on the journal you submit to. Assuming this manuscript is not a one-off episode, if you want to carry on and build on your research, you need to start the next project. Manuscript writing is a skill, which will improve the more you do it. As with any skill, you will find the better you get at it, the more you start to enjoy it. Once you become an experienced researcher, be sure to pass on your experience to the more junior researchers. For surgeons, writing your first manuscript can seem a daunting prospect and it is always nice to have a friendly senior researcher to guide you through the process.

References

1. Stroup DF, Berlin JA, Morton SC, et al. Meta-analysis of observational studies in epidemiology: a proposal for reporting. Meta-analysis Of Observational Studies in Epidemiology (MOOSE) group. JAMA. 2000;283(15):2008–12.
2. Moher D, Liberati A, Tetzlaff J, et al. Preferred reporting items for systematic reviews and meta-analyses: the PRISMA statement. BMJ. 2009;339:b2535.
3. von Elm E, Altman DG, Egger M, et al. The Strengthening the Reporting of Observational Studies in Epidemiology (STROBE) statement: guidelines for reporting observational studies. Lancet. 2007;370(9596):1453–7.
4. Schulz KF, Altman DG, Moher D, et al. CONSORT 2010 statement: updated guidelines for reporting parallel group randomised trials. BMJ. 2010;340:c332.

Chapter 14
Grant Writing

Dimitrios Stefanidis

Research grants provide the necessary means to successfully complete research projects. They are awarded to qualified individuals planning competitive projects and may significantly impact a surgeon's promotion and academic advancement. In this chapter, recommendations for a competitive grant application will be provided.

General Considerations

The search for a grant should begin with a project, a plan, and permission. Having a project in mind and identifying a suitable funding agency works generally better than the reverse (i.e. identifying a request for proposals and then creating a project). While several investigators will have their own research ideas upon which to base their grant proposal, a good approach to generate project ideas is to assess the needs of the applicant's field and brainstorm ideas with colleagues to identify important research questions needed to move

D. Stefanidis, M.D., Ph.D., F.A.C.S. (✉)
Department of Surgery, Indiana University,
545 Barnhill Drive; Emerson Hall 125, Indianapolis,
Indiana, 46202, USA
e-mail: dimstefa@iupui.edu

© Springer International Publishing AG 2017
D.B. Renton et al. (eds.), *The SAGES Manual Transitioning to Practice*, DOI 10.1007/978-3-319-51397-3_14

the field forward. A good knowledge of the available literature on the topic that can be accomplished via a comprehensive literature review will help refine initial ideas and research questions. Developing a research plan and determining its feasibility is the immediate next step. Obtaining input early from a statistician to define the best methodological approach to the study is imperative to avoid headaches later. Considering the available institutional resources and personnel, the time commitment and effort required from the investigator, and the required funding will help determine the feasibility of the project. Applicants should consider their strengths and weaknesses and pursue strategic partnerships that will offer them necessary expertise when lacking. Identifying the individuals who will be needed to conduct the study and winning their buy-in and support may be important for the success of the project. Identifying a research mentor is perhaps the single most important factor for success. Experienced mentors can be an invaluable resource that can guide the applicant in every step of the process.

Becoming familiar with the institution's regulatory requirements and deadlines and obtaining necessary permissions (i.e. IRB or IACUC approvals, support letters, etc.) will make the process more seamless and minimize surprises. Determining an appropriate budget for the proposed work is of paramount importance to ensure the necessary resources will be available to successfully conduct the project once funded. Poor attention to the budget can threaten the feasibility of the study. Given that most applicants in their early career have limited understanding of research budgets, help from experienced personnel in the grants and contracts office should be pursued early.

During this process, the applicant should also identify the appropriate funding agency with an interest in the research topic. Early communications with responsible agency representatives will help determine if funding is available and whether the project is of interest to the agency. It is helpful to obtain prior successful applications for review, if available, to use as guides when putting the grant proposal together. Any potential institutional research funding opportunities should be explored first. The competition for these seed grants is typically significantly lower than for external grants and thus the likelihood of success higher. Novice applicants will only gain valuable experience by pursuing such funding opportunities. Furthermore, pilot data are usually necessary when competing for larger external grants and can be obtained by using seed funding from the applicant's institution.

Once the potential funding opportunity has been identified, the applicant should carefully review the submission deadline and assess whether the available time frame is adequate.

Having a realistic picture of the time and effort required to prepare the application and to complete the project is imperative. In general, it takes about 1 year to collect pilot data, 1–2 months for IRB and/or IACUC approval, and 1–3 months to write the grant. The grant review may take 5–6 months from the submission deadline and up to 9 months to receive a funding decision.

Writing a Competitive Grant

First and foremost, the applicant should become familiar with the submission guidelines of the funding agency and observe them strictly. Not following these guidelines is an easy and almost guaranteed way to get your application rejected. While different funding agencies may use different application formats, grant sections typically required by most agencies are abstract/project summary, background and significance, preliminary work, hypothesis and specific aims, research design and methods, budget, assurances, available resources, and investigator curriculum vitae.

Abstract/Project Summary

This section describes succinctly every important aspect of the proposal with the exception of the budget and is usually limited to half or one page. It is a very important part of the application as it is used in the grant referral process and may be the only aspect of the application that is reviewed by non-primary reviewers to understand the proposal. It should include a brief background, the specific aims or hypotheses, unique features of the project, methodology (action steps) to be used, expected results, evaluation methods, a description of how the results will affect other research areas, and the significance of the proposed research.

This section should be brief but complete, clear, and enticing. Use all the allotted space and write this section last to reflect the entire proposal. This section should be viewed as a one-page advertisement for the project. This gives the first impression to the reviewers and should be constructed very carefully. While you can't win the grant on the first page, you can lose it!

Background, Significance, and Rationale

The background and significance section supports why it is worth conducting and funding the proposal. This section should include the problem to be investigated, the rationale for the proposed research, a critical, focused literature review and identification of knowledge gaps, and how the results of the proposed study will fill those gaps. A compelling argument should be presented for the importance and necessity of the proposal, the strong points (innovation, new strategies, etc.) of the proposal should be stressed, and the broader applicability of the study findings highlighted. An in-depth understanding of the relevant existing literature is necessary to demonstrate expertise in the topic and support the need for the proposed work. Acknowledgement of the work of others in the field is important, as they may be reviewers of your application.

Preliminary Results/Pilot Work

This section affords applicants the opportunity to demonstrate their experience and competence in conducting research projects and establish the feasibility and importance of the project. By describing the accumulated experience in the relevant topic, applicants demonstrate that they have the necessary skills to conduct the proposed project, and more importantly, that they can have confidence in their hypothesis. The critical preliminary findings that support the hypothesis and research design should therefore be included in this section. Prior successful, not directly related research work of the applicant can also help establish his/her competence. Lack of preliminary data will significantly weaken an application and its chances for funding. Given that accumulation of preliminary data can be very time-consuming, early planning is important.

Power Analysis/Sample Size Calculation

Power is the capability of a study to reliably detect any existing difference between study groups. Funding agencies recognize the risk of type II error with underpowered studies that may lead to wrong conclusions and threaten the validity of the study. A type II error occurs when a true difference exists between study populations, but there are insufficient numbers of subjects to detect this difference. Thus, by using a power analysis when designing studies, investigators can estimate the sample size needed to avoid erroneous interpretation of their results. Statistical support will help adequately address this section; importantly, sample size calculation may support or reject study feasibility early before too much effort has been invested in a particular project.

Hypothesis/Specific Aims

The purpose of this section is to provide a concise and realistic description of what the proposed research project is intended to accomplish. It begins with a description of the long-term goals of the study and states the hypothesis guiding the research. The hypothesis should be stated clearly, be testable, and adequately supported by the rationale and citations provided in the background section. Two to four specific and time-phased research aims should be provided. The specific aims should directly target the hypothesis, be related, and not interdependent in order to avoid all failing if one fails. Focus on aims supported by your expertise and pilot data and avoid losing focus by including an unrealistic hypothesis or citing too many aims.

Research Design and Methods

This section is crucial for the success of a proposal and describes how the research will be carried out. It will be reviewed very carefully and should include an overview of the experimental design and a detailed description of the specific methods that will be used to accomplish the specific aims of the study. A detailed discussion of how the results will be collected, analyzed, and interpreted is also required. Reference to study limitations, and potential pitfalls, and how these will be overcome with any alternative approaches should be included to demonstrate the investigator's thoughtfulness and maturity. A justification of why the chosen methodological approach is preferable to alternatives is necessary as well as the inclusion of controls when appropriate. The methods should be described in sufficient detail and succinctly and an algorithm of the research design should be included to aid reviewers' understanding and ease of reading. Publications in support of the application (preferably authored by the applicant) should be cited. The engagement of collaborators who supplement the applicant's expertise is strongly suggested. Finally, the inclusion of a timetable demonstrates thoughtful planning and organization and supports the feasibility of the project.

Budget and Justification

This section lists and provides justification for all expenses required to successfully complete the project's aims. The usual components include key and other personnel, consultants, equipment, supplies, travel, and other expenses. This is a very important aspect of the application and applicants should work closely with the institutional grants and contracts office when determining the budget. Having a good overview of the cost necessary to conduct the study will help the applicant decide which aspects of the proposal are feasible and which are not. A brief description of the duties for all proposed positions should be included, and the individuals for each position and their anticipated effort determined. In addition, a justification should be provided for equipment purchases and supply costs (detailed), project-related travel costs, and any included consultants or contractors. Being realistic and avoiding padding the budget or under-budgeting is important for the success of the proposal.

Assurances and Applicant Qualifications

Assurances are a necessary part of a grant proposal; they ensure that the applicant and institution will comply with all federal laws and regulations. It is best if Institutional Review Board and IACUC approvals are included in this section at the time of submission, but some agencies may allow the submission of these at a later time. A chairman's or appropriate institutional official's letter of support that guarantees protected time for the primary investigator and other key personnel during the study period is required. Letters of intent from collaborators should also be included. Demonstrating that the applicant can execute the proposed study and has adequate facilities and resources to complete the research is critical. The applicant should highlight his/her proposal-relevant contributions to the literature and achievements that support his/her role as a competent investigator. The reviewing process is very competitive and there will likely be several strong applicants in the pool. Therefore, this section needs to convey with facts that the applicant is the best possible individual to conduct the proposed study.

Overall Grantsmanship

Poor writing generally predisposes reviewers negatively to the proposed work. Therefore, the proposal should be succinct, visually stimulating, and easy to read and understand. Graphs and pictures should be used effectively to promote understanding. Avoiding jargon, spelling out acronyms, being consistent with terms, references, and writing style, and complying with the application's guidelines and format including adherence to the exact page allotment and specified type size are imperative. The application should be carefully proofread and checked for typos again and again. Have one or more colleagues who are knowledgeable and relevant to the field review your proposal prior to submission. The provided feedback will likely improve the proposal's clarity, and occasionally, may identify significant flaws the applicant may not have yet considered.

The Decision Is in: Now What?

If the decision letter is unfavorable, the applicant most likely will experience the five stages of grief (denial, anger, bargaining, depression, acceptance). Putting a grant together is a lot of work and having it be rejected leaves a very bad taste in your mouth. The last thing you should do, however, is give up. It takes time and dedication to get projects funded and, more often than not, the road to success is paved with failures. When you receive the rejection letter and critique, carefully review the reviewers' comments and determine if your design has any fatal flaws or is fixable. If the comments reflect enthusiasm about some aspects of the proposal and disappointment about others, it may mean that you are on the right path. The reviewers want typically to help applicants and will provide insight on how to improve the proposal, especially if they liked the idea but thought that the methodology was inadequate. If you think that the idea/research question is worth pursuing further after reviewing the comments, fix any identified problems, revise your proposal according to the guidance provided by the reviewers and resubmit to the same or a different appropriate agency. Do not forget to check back with your collaborators and get their input on how to proceed before resubmission; you may have to add some new collaborators to enhance your collective expertise based on comments received. If the reviewer's comments reflect lack of enthusiasm about the study idea and the innovation of the proposal, you may need to go back to the drawing board together with your research team.

If the grant is awarded, then besides organizing a big celebration, the real work of implementing the proposal begins. How well all aspects of the proposal had been thought out and budgeted for up front will become clear during this implementation. The execution of the proposal takes significant time and effort that the PI needs to ensure will be committed for the successful completion of the study. Regular research team meetings that monitor the achievement of the project's milestones in a timely manner and the budget expenditures are imperative for success. Any significant changes or issues should be communicated to the funding agency early and regular project updates provided. Importantly, enjoy the process and celebrate the products of your research for which you worked so hard.

Tips for Success and Common Pitfalls to Avoid

Tips

- Find a research mentor early
- Avoid dense sections in the proposal that are difficult to comprehend
- Be clear, concise, and succinct; the grant should be easy to read; avoid language/grammatical errors
- Do not overpromise what you cannot deliver

- Have a clear and realistic plan for your project and how you will accomplish your proposed aims, including how you are going to measure your project's success
- Propose a feasible and appropriate experimental design
- Proposal has the potential to lead to further studies or funding
- Be persistent and determined to succeed
- Demonstrate your maturity as a researcher by identifying potential problems or barriers and propose ways to prevent or overcome them if they occur during your study
- Convince reviewers that your study is absolutely necessary for the common good, has strong potential to advance the field, and that you have assembled the ideal team to take on the proposed project
- Seek help with the writing and submission process (advice, help, and criticism by seasoned grant writers, researchers, proofreaders, grants and contracts officials, etc.); involve a statistician early
- Seek collaboration with other researchers that will supplement your expertise by helping assemble a strong research team that can handle all aspects of the proposal
- Plan early, know all submission deadlines, and have a clear submission timeline so that submission-associated stress can be minimized and errors avoided
- Identify the most appropriate funders for the project (due diligence); research internal opportunities
- Timely acquisition of required assurances and support letters
- Create a realistic budget; avoid over- and underbudgeting
- Include graphs, images, or study algorithms as necessary to improve readability of your proposal

Pitfalls

- Lack of innovation of the research question/proposal
- Unclear research question and methodology
- Study aims not aligned with the funding agency goals and objectives

- Study aims lacking specificity and not being linked to methods
- Inappropriate study design that cannot answer the research question or an untestable hypothesis
- Weak rationale for your proposal
- Lack of preliminary results
- Not including a power analysis/sample size calculation where needed
- Incomplete applications; not following proposal guidelines
- Poor grantsmanship
- Overambitious proposal that lacks feasibility
- Inadequate expertise of research team for proposed study; limited collaboration
- Failure to include all relevant literature on the topic; failure to give credit to the work of the most prominent researchers in the field (which can be your reviewers!)

Chapter 15
The Application of Biostatistics to Your Surgical Practice

Vlad V. Simianu, Mark Pedersen, Rebecca P. Petersen, and Anjali S. Kumar

Introduction

As academic centers recruit and hire junior faculty to fill the large shoes of senior surgeons who are retiring or are promoted to new positions, the number of new responsibilities that are foreign to a recent graduate of a surgical training program can be overwhelming. In addition to being the

V.V. Simianu, M.D., M.P.H.
Surgical Outcomes Research Center, University of Washington, Seattle, WA, USA

Department of Surgery, University of Washington, Seattle, WA, USA

M. Pedersen, M.D.
Department of Surgery, University of Iowa Hospitals and Clinics, Iowa City, IA, USA

R.P. Petersen, M.D., M.S.
Department of Surgery, University of Washington, Seattle, WA, USA

A.S. Kumar, M.D., M.P.H. (✉)
Department of Surgery, Virginia Mason Medical Center, Seattle, WA, USA
e-mail: askumarmd@gmail.com

© Springer International Publishing AG 2017　　　　　217
D.B. Renton et al. (eds.), *The SAGES Manual Transitioning to Practice*, DOI 10.1007/978-3-319-51397-3_15

primary point-person of complex patient panels, young surgeons also juggle medical record upkeep, billing, and practice promotion. Those who land jobs with academic appointments may be asked to perform and publish research. Productivity in these arenas may influence the new faculty member's ability to rise in rank over the years, thus affecting salary.

Even when/if the position is exempt from performing research, teaching faculty will be asked to participate and/or lead journal review conferences for the department or section. An intelligent and insightful review of the literature selected can make an indelible impression on a colleague in the community. Arrive prepared to discuss the studies that have been selected by using this chapter and its pearls (Fig. 15.1) as your primer to the daunting, but decipherable, world of biostatistics.

What Is the Study's Purpose?

A study's purpose drives the selection of data sources, outcomes of interest, study design, and analytic plan. In general, the purpose of a study falls into two categories: hypothesis-generating or hypothesis-testing. Hypothesis-generating (sometimes called descriptive) studies aim to identify possible associations and motivate future investigations. Hypothesis-testing studies should make clear whether the hypothesis concerns superiority, inferiority, or equivalence (non-inferiority), and every attempt to exclude the influence of chance and bias in evaluating the hypothesis.

To succinctly summarize the research question that a study aims to address, we recommend that the discussant uses the "PICOT framework:" Population, Intervention (i.e., independent variables, exposure, and covariates), the Comparator group (if applicable), Outcome (i.e., dependent variable or endpoint), and Time frame of outcomes assessment [1–3]. Approaching research studies through a PICOT lens can guide the reader/reviewer systematically through the pertinent considerations when appraising the work.

- The research question can be succinctly summarized using the "PICOT" framework (Population, Intervention, Comparator group, Outcome, and Time frame)
- Recognizing of the minimal-clinically important difference (or MCID) for a particular patient-reported outcome (PRO) is helpful to help the reader distinguish between results that are significant statistically and those which are perceived as clinically significant to patients.
- ITT (intention to treat) analysis is essential because it provides information about how the intervention compares at the moment the decision is being made and is particularly useful at counseling patients.
- If the data are skewed (not normally distributed) the mean will be a biased estimator of the central tendency. In these cases, the median provides a better estimate.
- As a general rule, the larger the difference being compared and the larger the sample size for a given comparison, the lower the p value, and the less likely that the finding is the result of chance alone.
- When multiple comparisons are necessary, corrections (e.g., Bonferonni correction) to appropriately lower the p-value can be made in an attempt to safeguard against Type I errors (a false-positive finding).
- *Type II error* (a false-negative finding) most commonly occurs when a study has insufficient power (insufficient size) to detect true differences in outcomes between groups.
- When the summary measure is the absolute difference or relative risk, a CI inclusive of 0 indicates no statistically significant difference. If the summary measure is an odds ratio, a CI inclusive of 1.0 indicates no statistical difference in outcomes.
- When the continuous variable is not normally distributed, an alternative to the t-test, such as the Wilcoxon rank-sum test, may be more appropriate
- Fisher's exact test is more appropriate for such comparisons when the sample size is small (<100).
- As a rule of thumb, a minimum of 10 events (and equivalent number of nonevents) per variable are required for logistic regression (binary outcome) and 10 to 15 observations per variable for linear regression (continuous outcome).
- Odds ratio will overestimate the probability if the outcome occurs frequently (>10%) in the population.

Fig. 15.1 Pearls: tips and tricks for deciphering statistical implications of studies

Is the Right Data Being Used?

Many sources of information exist to conduct clinical research, and the selection of a data source is driven by a balance between the study purpose, resources (i.e., money), and feasibility (i.e., acceptance, ethics, and time). Table 15.1—Data sources provides a synopsis of commonly used data sources. The strengths and limitations of each are highlighted. For example, many datasets rely completely on administrative data (i.e., Medicare claims). These datasets are readily available to researchers and relatively inexpensive to obtain and analyze. However, they only reliably include metrics related to the billable aspects of care.

What Is the Measured Outcome?

Outcomes assessment cannot determine which intervention is better for the patient, but it can inform patients and providers about differences between competing diagnostic or therapeutic options. It is therefore important to determine which outcomes were assessed in a study, from what perspective, and whether these were consistent with the study's purpose. Outcomes may be subjective (e.g., patient satisfaction) or objective (e.g., death). There are categories of outcomes that the study designer or evaluator should be familiar with: (1) clinical outcomes, (2) patient-reported outcomes (PROs), (3) financial outcomes.

Clinical outcomes are well-defined, validated, and relatively easy to measure. Those related to in-hospital safety (safety outcomes) only require a short follow-up period. Operative mortality and postoperative complications (morbidity) are the most commonly measured safety endpoints. While, fortunately, mortality and complications tend to be infrequent events, the statistical implications are that safety studies often need to be quite large in sample size to be able to identify differences. One approach to address the costs of large samples or long lag times of development of infrequent

TABLE 15.1 Common data sources and their unique advantages and disadvantages (adapted, with permission, from Simianu et al. [17])

Data source	Advantages	Disadvantages	Example
Medical records	Easy to obtain Useful for hypothesis generation	Missing data Time-consuming Inability to measure certain information (e.g., intent) Limited scientific value	Case reports Case series
Patient-Reported Outcomes (PRO)	Unique data on symptoms, function, and health status Global (multidimensional) or Specific (unidimensional)	Time-consuming: interviews or questionnaires Unique instruments can have validity issues when population broadened Change/effect can be difficult to interpret	SF-36 Health Survey Patient-Reported Outcomes Measurement Information System (PROMIS)
Registry	Often contains clinical data Population-based real-world data not restricted to tertiary or referral centers	Built for limited reasons, so has restricted data Often has missing data because information captured from usual care rather than research visits Often include only cross-sectional data and need linkage to other data sources for follow-up	SEER National Cancer Database Device registries (Transcatheter Aortic Valve Replacement, TAVR)

(continued)

TABLE 15.1 (continued)

Data source	Advantages	Disadvantages	Example
National surveys	National sample Some longitudinal diagnoses and health care claims data	May over-represent certain racial groups in survey sample	Medical expenditure panel survey
Quality Improvement and Surveillance Project	Prospectively collected data Rich in clinical, laboratory, and demographic patient data	Overrepresentation of tertiary or referral centers Only a random sample of patients, not comprehensive	National Surgical Quality Improvement Project Society of Thoracic Surgeons database
Administrative	Large numbers Real-world data Often generalizable Easy to obtain Affordable	Limited clinical variables Data collected for billing, not research	Medicare State discharge data
Linked datasets	Richer source of data than either registry or administrative alone Allows longitudinal assessment of episodes of care	Missing data Inability to capture intent of therapy	SEER-Medicare

SEER surveillance, epidemiology, and end results program

clinical events is to report *surrogate endpoints*. Surrogate endpoints are intermediate outcomes that might serve as a surrogate for the actual clinical effect. However, the reader must consider whether the selected outcome is a meaningful clinical endpoint or simply a more easily measured surrogate [4]. Alternatively, when events are rare or there is no single optimal outcome, studies may report *composite endpoints*. For composite endpoints to be meaningful, however, they should be of similar importance and frequency. Imbalance in the components will not allow reviewers to judge which individual outcome contributed most to the composite endpoint.

Patient-reported outcomes (PROs) measure experiences or events that are reported by the patient. Sometimes, PROs are regarded as subjective outcomes because the response cannot be verified by a provider or researcher. Examples of common PRO concepts are health-related quality of life (HRQOL), satisfaction with care, functional status, well-being, and health status. Discrete concepts (PRO domains), include physical (e.g., pain), psychological (e.g., depression), and social functioning (e.g., the ability to carry out activities of daily living). Researchers are advised to use existing instruments to measure PROs (rather than creating their own) because the appropriate development of a questionnaire requires significant time, resources, testing, and validation before application. Recognition of the minimal-clinically important difference for a particular PRO distinguishes between results that are significant statistically and those which are perceived as clinically significant to patients [5].

Increasingly, *financial outcomes* are being added to contemporary studies. In these scenarios, it is important to note the difference between charges (the amount of money requested for health services and supplies) and costs (the actual amount of money spent). In addition, it is important to recognize that handling cost data requires special statistical approaches because costs are highly skewed (a few patients experience disproportionately higher costs than the majority) and exist as point masses (where many patients incur no costs). As an alternative to cost data, some authors report resource utilization which can range from pre-hospital resources (such as clinic visits and preoperative tests) to hospital resources (length of stay, readmissions, pharmacy services) to post-hospital care (skilled nursing facilities and home care). Similar to cost data, resources utilization data suffers from skewing and clustering. Three common approaches to cost-outcomes are cost-benefit, cost-utility, and cost-effectiveness analyses.

What Is the Hypothesis Being Tested?

Hypothesis testing is used to determine whether observed differences between two or more groups are true findings or are attributable to chance alone. Prior to testing a hypothesis, it is important to first define the null and alternative hypotheses. A *null hypothesis* is the principle that there is no difference among groups. The *alternative hypothesis* is the idea that there is a difference among two groups. A researcher needs to know with an acceptable level of accuracy whether an outcome is occurring due to the alternative hypothesis being correct or by chance alone. The p-value is a statistical summary measure for hypothesis testing and is interpreted as the probability that the observed difference in outcomes between groups is the result of chance (i.e., the difference is not actually based on the effect of the intervention). A significant level of 5% ($p = 0.05$) is widely accepted in medical literature to indicate a statistically significant finding. This threshold is rather arbitrary and for some measures a lower (large databases where false positive are to be avoided) or higher level (when a higher noise-to-signal ratio is acceptable as in safety evaluations) may be appropriate. As a general rule, the larger the difference being compared and the larger the sample size for a given comparison, the lower the p-value, and the less likely that the finding is the result of chance alone.

There are two types of errors which can occur with any hypothesis testing. Understanding how to address them is pertinent to the study purpose, design, and analytic plan. A *type 1 error* or *false positive* occurs when one observes a difference in outcomes when one does not actually exist. In this case, the null hypothesis is incorrectly rejected. For example, if a threshold of 5% ($p < 0.05$) were considered statistically significant, 5 of 100 statistical tests could potentially demonstrate a statistically significant finding that is attributable to chance alone. If one repeats a comparative analysis in different subgroups (i.e., multiple comparisons), then there are more opportunities to observe a false-positive result. When multiple comparisons are necessary, corrections (e.g., Bonferonni correction) to appropriately lower the p-value can be made in an attempt to safeguard against type I errors. A *type II error* occurs when no difference in outcomes is observed when a difference truly exists (a *false-negative* finding). That is to say, the null hypothesis was inappropriately accepted as correct. This type of error most commonly occurs when a study has insufficient power (insufficient size) to detect true differences in outcomes between groups.

Hypothesis testing can also be performed by examining confidence intervals (CI) of summary measures. Often the difference between groups are provided as an estimated ratio (in the study group divided by the control group) or as an absolute difference, with a 95% CI. The CI provides an estimate of the uncertainty around a given value. A wide CI suggests a lack of precision and a tight (small) interval indicates minimal uncertainty. When the summary measure is the absolute difference or relative risk, a CI inclusive of 0 indicates no statistically significant difference. If the summary measure is an odds ratio, a CI inclusive of 1.0 indicates no statistical difference in outcomes.

The power of a given study is the probability of rejecting the null hypothesis when it is in fact false. In more simple terms, power is a study's ability to find an association between two variables if one exists. Power is a value calculated based on a fixed and known sample size. Power is based on both study sample size and magnitude of difference observed or predicted in the dependent (response) variable in response to the independent variable. Power analysis should be done prior to completing any statistical analysis of a study and a reasonable power for a study is widely regarded as 0.8. If the power of a study is not found to be acceptable, the reverse calculation can be made to determine a necessary sample size to determine a statistical association. Power analysis is often required for grant funding for experimental research study designs. Retrospective studies of clinical or epidemiological data with large sample sizes seldom have a preliminary power analysis.

What Are the Implications of the Study Design That Was Chosen?

Several study designs are commonly used in surgical research and depend on the study purpose (hypothesis-generating versus hypothesis-testing) and the feasibility and resources for conducting the research. A synopsis of the most common study designs in surgical literature is provided in Table 15.2 – Study designs.

Randomized controlled trials (RCTs) provide the highest level of evidence supporting causality. Subjects are randomly assigned to an intervention group, where they receive an experimental intervention or to a control group, where they receive a controlled measurable alternative. If the number of randomized individuals is sufficiently large and randomization is performed properly, confounding variables will be distributed equally between groups and outcomes can be compared without concern for bias. However, conducting an RCT is challenging because of issues concerning equipoise, ethics, willingness to be randomized, costs, and generalizability.

An important analytic issue with RCTs is *intent-to-treat* (ITT). When an analysis is conducted following the ITT principle, outcome comparisons between control and treatment groups are based on the initial randomization and disregard subjects who cross over across intervention arms. If analytic approaches other than ITT are used, an equal balance of confounders across comparison groups cannot be guaranteed,

TABLE 15.2 Important considerations in design types

Study type	Exposure/outcome relationship	Considerations
Randomized controlled trial[T]	Randomly assigned an exposure and followed for outcome	Equipoise? Choice of control (placebo vs. standard of care) Generalizability? Blinding? Intention to treat? Superiority versus non-inferiority
Cross-sectional[T,G]	Exposure and outcome are assessed at the same point in time	Not suitable if disease has short duration or is rare
Cohort[T,G]	Identified by exposure, followed for outcome (prospective or retrospective)	One exposure, multiple outcomes Confounding Inefficient for rare outcomes or those which occur long after exposure
Case–control[T,G]	Identified by outcome, assessed for exposure (prospective or retrospective)	One outcome, multiple exposures How was control group chosen? Confounding Recall bias
Case report, series[G]		Generalizability

Adapted from Rosenthal et al. [3]
Can be considered hypothesis-testing (T) and/or hypothesis-generating (G)

and the benefits of randomization may be lost. ITT analysis is essential because it provides information about how the intervention compares at the moment the decision is being made and is particularly useful at counseling patients. When considering whether the patient should undergo a particular intervention, neither the patient nor the surgeon knows whether the patient will be able to complete the intervention strategy or will require another approach. Instead, the ITT will communicate the intended benefit for recommending a particular intervention.

While any one study may be underpowered to answer a given research question, *meta-analysis* is a technique that pools available published data in an effort to increase the statistical power of an analysis. Meta-analysis can be applied to RCT data or observational studies. Readers should consider that guidelines have been developed to ensure the quality and validity of results obtained through RCTs, the Consolidated Standards of Reporting Trials (CONSORT) [6, 7] and meta-analysis, the QUOROM (Quality of Reporting of Meta-Analyses) [8] and MOOSE (Meta-Analysis of Observational Studies in Epidemiology) [9] meta-analysis. Regardless of the type of pooled data, in all cases, an important consideration in appraising a meta-analysis is the homogeneity of the pooled studies. Significant heterogeneity indicates more variation in study outcomes than chance alone can explain. This is particularly a concern when observational data have been aggregated because these studies tend to have less control of variability and minimal control of confounding and bias. One approach to increasing the transparency of pooled results from observational studies is to also pool the baseline characteristics of the comparison groups.

Cross-sectional studies use data collected at a single point in time and are best used for hypothesis generation. This study design is commonly used to explore relationships between variables and disease burden though the data can be stacked over time to look at temporal trends. The main limitations arise from how a population is sampled and detection or recall bias.

Cohort studies follow patients non-randomly assigned to different groups to determine whether outcomes vary across groups. While cohort data may be captured prospectively or retrospectively, the onset of observation begins with the group assignment (i.e., exposure) and continues over time to determine whether a particular event occurred. Cohort studies are useful to estimate the rates (i.e., incidence) of exposures and outcomes, assess multiple outcomes, but are inefficient for evaluating outcomes that are rare, or occur a long time after exposure.

Case–control studies compare the frequency of exposures between patients who have and have not experienced an outcome of interest. These studies begin by enrolling subjects with and without the outcome of interest and then look back in time to search for differences in potential risk factors. Advantages of the case–control design include efficiency in evaluating the factors associated with rare outcomes or outcomes occurring a long time after exposure and the ability to evaluate multiple exposures simultaneously. Case–control designs are infrequently used in the surgical literature.

A *case report* or *series* aim to highlight an unusual or unexpected procedure or event. These studies propose a potential benefit or adverse effect of surgical therapy and may prompt more rigorous scientific evaluation. These studies are distinct from cohort investigations because there is no comparison made between competing strategies or interventions.

What Is the Variable Being Tested?

In simple terms, scientific investigation is the examination of variables. The first objective of a study is to identify the *independent* or *predictor* variable and the *dependent* or *response* variable. The dependent variable is that which changes in response to the independent variable. In experimental research, the independent variable can be manipulated to observe effects it has on the dependent variable. When it is not feasible to manipulate the independent variable for logistic, legal, or ethical reasons, nonexperimental studies attempt to show association between an independent and dependent variable through statistical inferences.

Categorical variables have discrete values and are typically described in proportions or frequencies. The simplest categorical variable is a *binary variable* that can only take on one of two values (i.e., yes/no). *Ordinal variables* are ordered categorical variables (i.e., ASA class). *Nominal variables* are unordered categorical variables (i.e., ethnicity). A *continuous variable* is one that can take on any number of values within a specified range of possibilities. Age is an example of a continuous variable. Descriptive statistics are used to describe the central tendency of continuous variables. The arithmetic mean provides a good estimate of central tendency for normally distributed (Gaussian or bell-shaped) data. If the data are skewed (not normally distributed), the mean will be a biased estimator of the central tendency. In these cases, the median or geometric mean provides a better estimate.

Time-to-event variables consist of two variables, a continuous variable that measures the time interval from an established start point (e.g., date of diagnosis or therapy) to a binary failure event (e.g., death or disease recurrence) or the end of the observation period. Time-to-event variables are typically reported as a probability of an event occurring at a certain point in time (i.e., survival at 5 years). Typically, time-to-event methods (the most commonly used is Kaplan-Meier) consider that number of patients at risk for an event decreases over time. Because of this, some methods may overestimate risk in the setting of competing risks (the disease evolves and prompts re-intervention; over time, a contraindication to re-intervention may develop, or death may occur, in which case a patient is no longer at risk). However, methods exist for handling time to event variables in the setting of competing risks [10].

Was the Correct Analysis Performed?

Central Tendency

The point at which observations tend to cluster is a frequent point of interest in scientific investigation. The mean, median, and mode of a group of observations each provide an assessment of this tendency and have their own practical uses. The *mean* is the summation of all observations for a given group of data divided by the number of observations in that data. The mean is highly sensitive to outlying observations within a dataset and can be an invalid assessment of central tendency if the data are skewed to one direction. The *median* is not as influenced by outlying observations and is defined as the observation at the 50th percentile for a group of observations. The third most commonly used and reported measure of central tendency is the *mode*, which is the set of values in a group of observations that occurs most frequently.

When considering a measure of central tendency, it is also important to consider the dispersion of the observations around the measure. The *range* of a group of measurements is the difference between the largest and smallest observation in a dataset and can give a crude assessment of the dispersion of observations. This value is again heavily influenced by outlying observations. The *variance* of a set of observations is the sum of squared distance from all observations to the mean in a given group of observations divided by 1-number of observations, and *standard deviation* is the square root of the variance. Standard deviation is the most widely reported assessment of dispersion due to its properties. For a relatively symmetric group of data, 67% of the observations will be within +/− one standard deviation from the mean and 95% of the observations will be within +/− two standard deviations from the mean. The 95% confidence interval of a mean is thus bounded by the values two standard deviations below and above the mean, respectively. Furthermore, a mean from one group of observations can be said to be significantly different from a mean of another set of observations if the 95% confidence intervals do not overlap.

Rates

Some demographic data describing a population can be reported through measures of central tendency such as age and BMI. Not all data can be reported using these measures. Many demographic variables such as gender, race, comorbidities, and behavioral attributes such as smoking must be reported as rates. Other vital statistics such as births, deaths, and disease prevalence and incidence are also reported as rates.

Probability

An extension of rates is probability. The relative risk (RR) is a comparison of probabilities. RR is the probability of an event such as death, disease, or complication in subjects with a given exposure compared to the probability of death, disease, or complication in subjects without this exposure. A relative risk of 1.0 would indicate that the risk for death among the diseased group would be identical to those without disease. The odds ratio is a comparison of the odds as opposed to the probability of an event. While probability is proportion of outcome of interest to all observations, odds are the outcome of interest in proportion to the alternative outcome. The odds of an event are not a risk or probability or risk per se. As such, it is a more appropriate statistic to compute in retrospective studies such as case–control or cross-sectional studies, where risk cannot be determined. In prospective cohort studies and RCTs, relative risk is an acceptable statistic.

It is important to note that the odds ratio will overestimate the probability if the outcome occurs frequently (>10%) in the population [11]. When the outcome is rare, the odds generally provide a good approximation of the probability. It is particularly relevant when conducting multivariable analysis that a minimum number of events are included to achieve a reliable estimate. As rules of thumb, a minimum of 10 events (and equivalent number of nonevents) per variable are required for logistic regression (binary outcome) [12] and 10–15 observations per variable for linear regression (continuous outcome) [13]. This should also be considered when multiple variables are being controlled for in a multivariable model.

Diagnostic Testing

Probability forms the basis for the value of a diagnostic test. The probability of disease given a test result is paramount to accurately diagnosing or ruling out disease in a patient. Multiple measures of probability are used to assess the accuracy of a given diagnostic test. The *sensitivity* of a test is the probability of a positive test given a patient has the disease being tested. Another assessment of accuracy is *specificity* which is the probability of a negative test given a patient does not have the disease. These are important measures of accuracy for establishing the usefulness of a screening tool. Many times an individual will wonder what the probability of disease is given they test positive or the probability that they don't have disease given a negative test result. These measures are the *positive* and *negative predictive values,* respectively. Positive and negative predictive values are heavily influenced by disease prevalence while sensitivity and specificity are not. As a result of this variation in diagnostic power, PPV and NPV are less favored to the positive and negative likelihood ratios as both of these tests can be calculated using sensitivity and specificity. The *positive likelihood ratio* can be calculated as (sensitivity)/(1-specificity) and the *negative likelihood ratio* can be calculated as (1-sensitivity)/(specificity). Positive and negative likelihood ratios greater than 10 and less than 0.1, respectively, offer significant shifts in likelihood of disease. Positive and negative likelihood ratios less than 2 and greater than 0.5, respectively, do not suggest significant impact on likelihood of diagnosis.

Statistical Testing

The *Student's t-test* is one of the most common tests for analyzing sample means. The *t*-test is based on null and alternative hypotheses. Notwithstanding the type of *t*-test being run, the null hypothesis is always that no difference exists. A one sample *t*-test is used to test if a sample mean is different from a known population mean. A two-sample t-test can be either paired or independent. A paired, two-sample t-test is used to test the difference between matched samples, such as the mean systolic blood pressure in patients before starting a drug and those same patients after 6 months on therapy. An independent, two sample t-tests are used to test the difference in sample means between two unrelated samples, such as the difference in mean systolic blood pressure between patients with diabetes and patients without. A one-sided t-test is used if it is known that the test sample will either be less than or greater than a reference point. A two-sided t-test is used if this is not necessarily known.

The Student's t-test is limited in its utility to two samples. If a study design calls for multiple samples such as repeated measurements on a sample group or sampling from more than two groups, repeatedly running the Student's t-test increases the chance of a type I error, or finding an association by chance. In this setting, *Analysis of Variance (ANOVA)* is a more appropriate test. The ANOVA as its name would suggest creates a test statistic from of the dispersion or variance of a variable. The term variance in this instance is referring to general dispersion of the sample data, rather than the variance value described above. For the ANOVA, the dispersion or variance is calculated using the sum of squares method, which is again beyond the scope of this chapter. This variance (dispersion) is partitioned into, or calculated for, all subjects within-groups and between-groups. In this way, a single test statistic termed the F-statistic can be used to effectively determine if the means of three or more groups are different from each other. The F-statistic also correlates to a probability that is determined from the F distribution and this probability is again, the p-value. In a one-way ANOVA, the variation in the response variable is attributed to a single factor, i.e., the difference of the different sample groups. For example, suppose a research team is interested in recurrence of Crohn's ileitis after surgery and the effects of multiple types of drugs on remission, such as budesonide, methotrexate, and infliximab. The different drug regimens a subject is taking is the source of variation. A two-way ANOVA can be done if there are two factors such as anti-inflammatory medications and diet routines that could potentially affect recurrence. The two-way ANOVA will give a statistic for both medications and diet and the interaction of these two factors. The important thing to remember with ANOVA is that it will not indicate which groups are significantly different from each other, only that there is significant variation by group. Two group means may be the same, statistically speaking, while only the third is significantly different. In this instance, a t-test may be used to determine which group mean is different. However, it is important to again state that running multiple t-tests will raise the likelihood of a type I error. This can be overcome by lowering the threshold for significance below 0.05–0.01 or even lower. Additionally, multivariable methods can be employed to determine the individual group effects on the response variable.

The above tests are designed to assess the differences in group means. Often times, a study doesn't collect data that can be reported as a mean. As described above, the response variable is a yes or a no, disease or no disease, complication or no complication. Also, as described above, this can be described in terms of probability, risk, and odds. An alternative means of assessing categorical data of this nature is the *chi-square test*. The chi-square test makes use of contingency tables which, in their simplest form, are 2 × 2 tables with dichotomous dependent and independent variables. A 2 × 2 table could be constructed for patients who undergo cholecystectomy. Columns are patients who underwent either laparoscopic or open procedures and rows are bile leak versus no bile leak. The odds ratio or relative risk could be calculated in this instance. The chi-square test can also tell if the rate of bile leak is different between the two procedure types. The benefit of the chi-square test is that it can be extended to categorical data with more than two responses. For example, rates of bile leak could be compared to ASA class which has six responses. The chi-square test can be used to determine if rates of bile leak are increased based for patients with higher

ASA classifications. The chi-square test again utilizes a test statistic calculated based on the observed and expected counts for each cell in the contingency table and a p-value is obtained from the chi-square distribution. A test called McNemar's test can be employed when data are paired.

Regression is a tool that is useful predicting response from some predictor variable. There are multiple regression methods that can be applied to different variable types. A *simple linear regression* is the most basic example and can be used when the response variable and predictor variable are continuous. For example, blood pressure changes with changes in subject age can be evaluated in this way. Regression makes use of the variation in response variables as they relate to the dependent variable. Another way to say this is, it uses the average of the response variable when the predictor value is fixed (i.e., the BP ranges for patients at age 35). If this average changes significantly when the predictor variable is changed, the predictor variable is a significant predictor of the response variable. Mathematics is unimportant as they are typically done by statistical analysis programs. With that said, a *p*-value is obtained that gives the probability that the variation in response due to the predictor is seen by chance. *Multivariable linear regression* can be utilized when there are multiple predictor variables being assessed. This is not to be confused with multivariate regression which is used for multiple response or dependent variables. Regression can also be performed on dichotomous or categorical outcome variables. In this instance, the logistic regression model is used. The logistic regression model will also provide a p-value for the association between the predictor and response but it will also provide an odds ratio for the given predictor variable.

All of the above tests rely on multiple assumptions for their validity. One of the most significant assumptions is that the parameter, or numerical characteristic of the population from which the study sample is drawn, fits a specified distribution. Typically, the assumption is a normal distribution. The central limit theorem makes this assumption true for most variables. However, this is not always the case. Nonparametric tests do not require this assumption, but have similar procedures to the above tests making use of other statistics such as the median. The *Wilcoxon Rank Sum* is the nonparametric equivalent of the Student's *t*-test and makes use of group medians rather than means and the *Kruskal–Wallis test* is the nonparametric equivalent of the ANOVA. Additionally, data transformations can be done, such as log(Variable) or ln(Variable) that can give the sample data a normal distribution. The decision to transform data and the method of transformation should be decided on during the design phase of a study and not part of post hoc analysis.

Table 15.3 summarizes the types of tests according to the categories of variables used.

How to Interpret the Study Findings?

One of the most important issues to consider in the evaluation and conduct of outcomes research, especially when observational data is being used, is *confounding*. A confounder is a measured or unmeasured variable associated with the exposure of interest and associated with the outcome. This dual relationship can influence the degree and direction of, or even completely mitigate, an observed association between exposure and outcome [14]. RCTs can address confounding through randomization. On the other hand, investigators who perform observational studies must address confounding both with analytical approaches (i.e., multivariable regression and propensity scores), and acknowledge potential residual confounding in their discussion of the study's limitations, noting variables that were not measured, their relationship with the exposure and the outcome, and their implication on the potential direction and magnitude of confounding bias.

It is important to consider the many forms of bias when evaluating research. For instance, there any many forms of selection bias which can favor administration of a particular intervention to those thought to need it the most. *Propensity score* analysis is an alternative method of risk adjustment to

TABLE 15.3 Summary of statistical testing by variable type

| Outcome→ | Continuous | Categorical | | |
| Exposure↓ | | Dichotomous | Ordinal | Polychotomous |
				Nominal
Continuous Univariate	Pearson Correlation Linear regression *Spearman rank correlation*	Logistic regression Discriminant analysis *Wilcoxon rank sum*	Ordinal regression *Spearman rank correlation*	Discriminant analysis *Kruskal–Wallis*
Multivariate	Multiple linear regression	Logistic regression Discriminant analysis	Ordinal regression	Discriminant analysis Nominal regression
CATEGORICAL **Dichotomous** Univariate	*t*-test ANOVA Linear regression *Wilcoxon rank sum*	Chi-square Logistic regression	*Wilcoxon rank sum* Chi-square test for trend Ordinal regression	Chi-square
Multivariate	*N*-way ANOVA Analysis of covariance Multiple linear regression	Mantel–Haenszel Logistic regression	Ordinal regression	Discriminant analysis Nominal regression

Matched	Matched pairs *t*-test	McNemar's test (univariate) Conditional logistic regression (multivariate)	Does not exist	Does not exist
Polychotomous ordinal or nominal Univariate	ANOVA Linear regression *Spearman rank correlation (ordinal)* *Kruskal–Wallis (nominal)*	Chi-square Logistic regression *Spearman rank correlation (ordinal)*	Chi-square test for trend Ordinal regression *Spearman rank correlation*	Chi-square Discriminant analysis Nominal regression
Multivariate	N-way ANOVA Multiple regression	Logistic regression	Ordinal regression	Chi-square Discriminant analysis Nominal regression
Matched	Repeated measures ANOVA *Multiple linear regression*	Conditional logistic regression	Does not exist	Does not exist

Italic text = nonparametric tests

reduce the bias in estimating treatment effects when analyzing nonrandomized, observational data. Because patients receiving one treatment tend to be different than patients receiving another (e.g., minimally invasive [MIS] as compared with open surgery), a propensity score is calculated using logistic regression to determine a subject's probability of having the exposure of interest (propensity to undergo MIS). The outcomes of interest for patients who do and do not undergo MIS (but have a similar propensity to undergo MIS) can then be compared through matching, stratified analyses, or regression (adjusting only for propensity) [15].

While propensity score analysis cannot adjust away all confounders, known or unknown, as these are intrinsic to observational data. However, there are three circumstances in which the use of propensity scores may be appropriate: (1) there are many confounders relative to the number of events (i.e., less than ten events per covariate) resulting in an unpowered regression analysis; (2) there is no interest in the association between the adjustment factors and outcome; and (3) the relationship between the exposure and propensity for treatment can be estimated more accurately than the relationship between the exposure and outcome [16].

Generalizability refers to the application of research findings to routine, clinical practice. While RCTs provide the highest level of evidence about the efficacy of competing interventions, they are conducted in a highly controlled environment, limiting other providers' ability to reproduce the delivery of care and outcomes in a non-research setting. In addition, generalizability issues apply to observational studies as well. Critical readers should consider why care patterns and outcomes described in research studies might not be reproducible in other clinical settings and patient populations.

Conclusions

Although not all jobs in surgery require academic productivity in the form of original clinical research, a basic familiarity with data sources, study design, and statistical testing can greatly enhance a young surgeon's ability to intelligently contribute to discussions involving the scientific literature. Early in our careers, this proficiency can manifest in many beneficial ways that stretch well beyond the surgical journal club setting: engaging our peers in multidisciplinary conferences, incorporating evidence-based principles into our own practices, volunteering to adjudicate scientific abstracts for society meetings, and providing peer-review for editorial boards, to name a few. We encourage you to approach any review with these five questions in mind: (1) What is the study's purpose? (2) Is the right data being used? (3) What is the measured outcome? (4) What are the implications of the study design that was chosen? (5) Was the correct analysis performed (and adequately powered to support the conclusion)?

References

1. Richardson WS, Wilson MC, Nishikawa J, Hayward RS. The well-built clinical question: a key to evidence-based decisions. ACP J Club. 1995;123(3):A12–3.
2. Schardt C, Adams MB, Owens T, Keitz S, Fontelo P. Utilization of the PICO framework to improve searching PubMed for clinical questions. BMC Med Inform Decis Mak. 2007;7:16.
3. Rosenthal R, Schafer J, Briel M, Bucher HC, Oertli D, Dell-Kuster S. How to write a surgical clinical research protocol: literature review and practical guide. Am J Surg. 2014;207(2):299–312.
4. Fleming TR, Powers JH. Biomarkers and surrogate endpoints in clinical trials. Stat Med. 2012;31(25):2973–84.
5. Jaeschke R, Singer J, Guyatt GH. Measurement of health status. Ascertaining the minimal clinically important difference. Control Clin Trials. 1989;10(4):407–15.
6. Turner L, Shamseer L, Altman DG, Weeks L, Peters J, Kober T, et al. Consolidated standards of reporting trials (CONSORT) and the completeness of reporting of randomised controlled trials (RCTs) published in medical journals. Cochrane Database Syst Rev. 2012;11:MR000030.
7. Nagendran M, Harding D, Teo W, Camm C, Maruthappu M, McCulloch P, et al. Poor adherence of randomised trials in surgery

to CONSORT guidelines for non-pharmacological treatments (NPT): a cross-sectional study. BMJ Open. 2013;3(12):e003898, 2013–003898.

8. Moher D, Cook DJ, Eastwood S, Olkin I, Rennie D, Stroup DF. Improving the quality of reports of meta-analyses of randomised controlled trials: the QUOROM statement. quality of reporting of meta-analyses. Lancet. 1999;354(9193):1896–900.

9. Stroup DF, Berlin JA, Morton SC, Olkin I, Williamson GD, Rennie D, et al. Meta-analysis of observational studies in epidemiology: a proposal for reporting. meta-analysis of observational studies in epidemiology (MOOSE) group. JAMA. 2000; 283(15):2008–12.

10. Resche-Rigon M, Azoulay E, Chevret S. Evaluating mortality in intensive care units: contribution of competing risks analyses. Crit Care. 2006;10(1):R5.

11. Chen W, Shi J, Qian L, Azen SP. Comparison of robustness to outliers between robust poisson models and log-binomial models when estimating relative risks for common binary outcomes: a simulation study. BMC Med Res Methodol. 2014;14:–82. doi:10.1186/1471-2288-14-82.

12. Peduzzi P, Concato J, Kemper E, Holford TR, Feinstein AR. A simulation study of the number of events per variable in logistic regression analysis. J Clin Epidemiol. 1996;49(12):1373–9.

13. Babyak MA. What you see may not be what you get: a brief, nontechnical introduction to overfitting in regression-type models. Psychosom Med. 2004;66(3):411–21.

14. Mehio-Sibai A, Feinleib M, Sibai TA, Armenian HK. A positive or a negative confounding variable? A simple teaching aid for clinicians and students. Ann Epidemiol. 2005;15(6):421–3.

15. Haukoos JS, Lewis RJ. The propensity score. JAMA. 2015;314(15):1637–8.

16. Austin PC. An introduction to propensity score methods for reducing the effects of confounding in observational studies. Multivar Behav Res. 2011;46(3):399–424.

17. Simianu VV, Farjah F, Flum D. Evidence-based surgery: critically assessing surgical literature (Chapter 8). In: Townsend CM, Beauchamp RD, Evers BM, Mattox KL, editors. Sabiston textbook of surgery. Philadelphia: Elsevier; 2016.

Index

© Springer International Publishing AG 2017
D.B. Renton et al. (eds.), *The SAGES Manual Transitioning to Practice*, DOI 10.1007/978-3-319-51397-3

CPSIA information can be obtained
at www.ICGtesting.com
Printed in the USA
BVOW07s1031070517
483430BV00008B/211/P